NORMAL PRESSURE HYDROCEPHALUS

A Guide for Doctors, Nurses, Patients, Families, Students, & Caregivers

JERRY BELLER HEALTH RESEARCH INSTITUTE

Copyright © 2019 Jerry Beller
All rights reserved.
ISBN-13: 9781701500495

DEDICATION

To people living with Dementia and their loved ones.

CONTENTS

FOREWORD 1

Who is the reading audience? 5

Two Dementia Series 14

I. DEMENTIA 16

Chapter 1: WHAT IS DEMENTIA? 17

Chapter 2: WHAT ARE THE 19 PRIMARY DEMENTIAS? 21

Chapter 3: WHO IS MOST LIKELY TO GET DEMENTIA? 23

Chapter 4: DEMENTIA COSTS & PREVALENCE 33

II. NORMAL PRESSURE HYDROCEPHALUS 46

Chapter 5: WHAT IS HYDROCEPHALUS? 47

III. NORMAL PRESSURE HYDROCEPHALUS SYMPTOMS 54

Chapter 6: NORMAL PRESSURE HYDROCEPHALUS SYMPTOMS (NPH) ...55

III. NORMAL PRESSURE HYDROCEPHALUS STAGES 60

Chapter 7: NORMAL PRESSURE HYDROCEPHALUS (NPH) STAGES 61

IV. NORMAL PRESSURE HYDROCEPHALUS RISK FACTORS 63

Chapter 8: NORMAL PRESSURE HYDROCEPHALUS RISK FACTORS 64

Age 65

V. DIAGNOSIS & TREATMENT 68

Chapter 9: HOW DO DOCTORS DIAGNOSE NORMAL PRESSURE

HYDROCEPHALUS?..69

    Chapter 10: TREATMENT FOR NORMAL PRESSURE HYDROCEPHALUS ...79

VI. BONUS SECTION 82

    Chapter 11: Starter To-do List for Somebody and Family once Diagnosed with Dementia. 83

CONCLUSION 96

THANK YOU FOR READING 100

BELLER HEALTH BOOKS 101

    Other Beller Health Books 104

ABOUT THE AUTHOR...105

ACKNOWLEDGMENTS

Thanks to the American Academy of Neurology, Atlanta Center for Medical Research, Alzheimer's Association, Alzheimer's Disease Center, Alzheimer's Disease Center of Northwestern University, Alzheimer's Foundation of America, American Academy of Neurology, Association for Frontotemporal Degeneration, Australia Neurological Research, CDC, Department of Health and Human Services, Duke University Medical Center, Emory Hospital, Harvard Medical School, Johns Hopkins Medicine, Mayo Clinic, National Aphasia Association, National Institute of Neurological Disorders and Strokes, National Library of Medicine, National Institute on Aging, National Institutes of Health, Prince of Wales Medical Research Institute, *PubMed*, Stanford Library School of Medicine, Stanford Medicine, UCSF Department of Neurology, UCSF Memory and Aging Center, University of Cambridge Neurology Unit, World Health Organization (WHO), *Journal of American Medical Association* (JAMA), and several other organizations that provided information used for this book. Thanks to everybody who assisted this book in a variety of important ways, and everybody at Beller Health Research Institute. To my editor, John Briggs, who helps me improve every book. To all sources and for the photos. Most of all, thanks to my wife, Nicola Beller

FOREWORD

Before diving into the book's subject matter, let's discuss two related Dementia series:

- *2020 Dementia Overview* series
- *2020 Dementia Types, Symptoms, Stages, & Risk Factors* series

2020 Dementia Overview series is an extension of the medical groundbreaking *19 Dementia Types, Symptoms, Stages, & Risk Factors* series, the first covering all primary dementia types.

After spending decades building an audience in other genres, including nutrition, circumstances turned the world upside down. Doctors diagnosed my mother with Alzheimer's. The same doctors soon diagnosed my father with cancer. A few months later, my father's favorite brother and my closest uncle died.

Three consecutive hard blows blew the world beyond recognition.

Tough and decent as they come, dad insisted on taking care of my mother while fighting brain cancer. My brothers and sister-in-law did their share, but Dad cared for my mother for a long time while they worked. Dad proved what a remarkable and great man he was down the stretch but finally succumbed to brain cancer.

My brothers and sister-in-law did their best to take care of mom, but it came at a price. Caregiving for a dementia patient is an indescribable horror I would not wish on my worst enemy.

You must watch somebody you love wilt away, little by little until dementia wipes away huge chunks of their personality.

Living away, my wife and I visited when possible. We saw how mom deteriorated, but also the effect caregiving had on my father and brothers. It was like watching a train wreck over and over, each time getting worse and helpless to prevent it.

Watching Alzheimer's takedown, my strong-willed mother and others bruised my soul. My writing shifted initially to learn about Alzheimer's, but the more learned, the more I cringed.

The cold hard facts rendered me speechless. Over 5.8 million Americans, and 44 million people worldwide, suffer Alzheimer's. No cure. Just a devastating and expensive slow march towards an agonizing end.

Not content to kill, Alzheimer's tortured Mom for years before killing her. It robbed her memory and damaged her brain, where she repeated herself in a continuous loop, each time thinking she was saying it the first time. As the disease advanced, the neurological disorder destroyed her mind and body.

Seeing dementia take down that tough old bird rattled me. While I could not bring back my mother, I dedicate my life to researching and writing about dementia 8-12 hours per day, six or seven days per week.

I tackled Alzheimer's to learn everything I could about the brute and determine how I and others might prevent it and other noncommunicable diseases. Having written on nutrition and advocated health in Washington, I already had a clue but determined to figure out how to prevent Alzheimer's. But I needed to know more, much more, about this terrorizing neurological disorder.

I learned Alzheimer's was just one of over one-hundred neurological disorders causing dementia. When I searched for a book covering the primary dementias, none existed. Instead, I turned to individual books and again found no books written on several of the most frequent dementias.

In what on the one hand seems like yesterday and the other a lifetime ago, I set out several years ago to write a dementia book covering the 15 most prevalent dementia types. The first to do that, I next wrote books covering each of the 15 most prevalent dementias.

In 2020, I expanded the book covering 15 dementias to 19 dementia types. I also released books on each of the 19 dementias. While proud of these medical firsts, I do not take myself too seriously.

As one of the dozens of scientists, neurologists, researchers, and writers who devote their lives to fighting the war against dementia, I remain humble. I appreciate the individual and combined accomplishments of everybody else in the field.

Nor should any of us get cocky knowing we're losing the war. If we win the war during my lifetime, I will celebrate with hundreds of people worldwide who helped defeat the great beast of our day.

My two-book series break medical ground, and I consider major achievements but remain two among hundreds of significant contributions to the dementia field by people around the globe.

The series provides patients and loved ones a great resource for dementias not covered as extensive as Alzheimer's and the more prevalent types.

By covering the 19 most prevalent dementias, doctors, nurses, and medical professionals benefit from a series covering neurological disorders causing 99% of dementia. The series helps primary care physicians, providers, and nurses who struggle to diagnose dementias with overlapping symptoms.

The series is an organic, evolving work, and each book receives major annual updates. As science uncovers information, we add important data in new editions. We also polish each edition.

We describe the writing goal in three ways:
1. Simplify the language and make it easier for nonscientists to comprehend.
2. Honor the science and facts.
3. Document science and include citations for doctors,

nurses, medical researchers, students, and patients.

Our goal is to provide invaluable medical information for professionals, patients, loved ones, and caregivers.

I do not reinvent the wheel but accumulate the best research and teach our readers a better understanding of Alzheimer's and the other 18 primary dementia types.

Among the worst news is one of our loved ones has dementia. A killer disease with no cure frightens the bravest souls.

This medical condition destroys, not just the inflicted, but their loved ones. Besides the patient, nobody suffers more than voluntary caregivers. Watching a mother, father, brother, sister, wife, or husband suffering dementia brutalizes the soul.

I study dementia year around to write and release annual updates to honor people—including my mother—taken by Alzheimer's or one of the other primary dementias.

Modest book royalties are the only compensation, as I accept no money from corporations to promote their product. Nor do I have an ax to grind with anybody in the medical profession.

Having written 100 plus books over four decades, I am thankful to readers for collectively providing me a decent income. However, now in my sixties, I care little about riches and fame.

Who is the reading audience?

The audience falls into five categories.

Those Diagnosed with Dementia

If doctors diagnose you with dementia, my heart goes out to you. You're in for a long battle. Do yourself a favor and focus on slowing the disease and extending the quality of life. One word of caution, the books in this series speak to not only patients, but also families, doctors, students, nurses, and caregivers. Many of those diagnosed with dementia appreciate and benefit from the books, but some find some of the material too disturbing. I intend to write books exclusively for patients but must finish the work related to this series first. While there is not anything too shocking, I wrote the material for a wide audience, meaning I am not always speaking to patients specifically. I promise to personalize an edition for patients and loved ones after finishing this series. By shining a light on all 19 primary dementia types, I hope to help the medical community better distinguish and diagnose neurological disorders.

Loved Ones of Those Diagnosed

If doctors diagnose a loved one with dementia, he or she needs you more than ever. Depending on the type, dementia causes behavioral problems, memory issues, motor decline, and other psychological and physical disorders. The learning curve is steep and changes as one moves from one stage to the next. As with those with dementia, I warn families these books provide a technical overview, and the emphasis is not always on the emotional aspect. If you want to learn about dementias, this series is a great option. If you're looking more for emotional support, there are more appropriate books. I also plan to write a book specifically for families once fulfilling responsibilities for this series.

Medical Professionals

If you are a medical professional interested in studying the dementias, the series covers the dementias responsible for 99% of dementia. While neurologists probably already know the 19 primary dementias, the books provide a quick overview and reference for primary care physicians, nurses, other medical professionals, and students. I also include citations so you can continue your investigation beyond the book's scope.

Volunteer & Professional Caregivers

If you are a dementia caregiver, you are also in for a long, difficult march. Dementia patients demand 24/7 care in later stages, requiring help to go to the bathroom, bathing, and other basic daily functions. While this series is not written solely for caregiving, caregivers benefit by gaining a better understanding of each dementia, their symptoms, and progression.

Anybody Wanting to Learn About A Disease That Strikes 1 Of 6 Americans, And 1 Of 3 Seniors

The series benefits anybody who wants to gain an intermediate understanding of the 19 dementias.

Series' First Lesson

Doctors, like teachers, are part of a sacred profession. **Nothing I say or write replaces your need for a competent doctor!** Nor does any criticism of the profession diminish my respect and admiration for the best.

I detest the worst teachers who fail students and society but love and respect the best. Society would crumble without the most devoted and competent teachers.

Similar, I abhor incompetent, greedy doctors who fail patients and society, but love and respect the best.

The profession must weed out incompetent, uncaring, corrupt doctors, and medical personnel. Every profession has a percentage of bad apples, but within the medical profession, they are cancerous!

Nothing good I write about the medical profession includes incompetent, uncaring doctors, researchers, nurses, etc. And nothing bad I write targets the best.

The series criticizes the profession when deserved, but the first lesson in this series: **Find a competent doctor!** If you have one, count your blessings. If not, find one.

Just as one can learn outside the classroom, we live in a blessed age where medical information is available for anybody on the internet. Such information serves us well, but do not—for a minute-think it replaces the need for a competent, devoted doctor.

The Wrong Doctors

Let me begin this section by saying I love and respect quality doctors, nurses, researchers, and medical professionals from the bottom of my heart and the fullness of my mind.

However, this section is not about what's right in the medical profession.

Glorified idiots, bad doctors are dangerous parasites who dishonor a noble profession. Smart enough to finish medical school, but greedy or flawed beyond redemption, they are like priests working for the devil. Among the worse members of society are doctors motivated by greed or limited by incompetence. Walking parasites!

The Wrong Doctors + Big Pharm + Big Insurance + Big Hospital = Expensive & Inadequate Health Care

Over the past few decades, Big pharmaceuticals, Big Insurance, and their political puppets appointed doctors sanctioned drug dealers. Entrusting the worse doctors with such powers produces little or no better results than assigning the task to a thug on the worst corner in America.

The worst doctors who hand out drugs like candy serve nobody's purpose but their own and Big Pharm.

Not an indictment of the entire profession, but unfortunately, Big Insurance dictates the typical office visit includes a quick examination and one or more prescriptions. The approach is not based on good science and runs counter to everything science teaches us.

What About Some Tough Love?

The one thing people today do not want is what we often need most, tough love. People want everything sugarcoated and easy.

The problem is most of the time; life is neither sweet nor easy.

What patients need much of the time is not an alleged "magic pill," but instead tough love. Doctors must learn nutrition and teach patients to eat healthier, exercise more, and get 7-8 hours of sleep per night. Like it or not, this is part of modern medicine. Showing up and passing out pills all day is not preventing Alzheimer's and other dementias, nor curing them.

Medical professionals must lead by example and embrace the science of nutrition, exercise, and sleep. If a healthy diet and exercise are the two cornerstones to health, the third is sleep.

The average person needs few or no drugs if they practice healthy habits.

Any doctor who does not vigorously advocate a balanced whole food diet, exercise most days of the week, and 7-8 hours' sleep per night neglects their duty and

Instead, too many doctors ignore the three cornerstones of health and are content to write their patients unnecessary and potentially dangerous prescriptions for the rest of their lives. 100% emphasis on treating symptoms with drugs, which often require more drugs to counter the side effects, is producing disastrous results. To be the best doctor, one must also emphasize prevention.

Failed Drug Trials

None of the drug trials have produced even one drug that cures Alzheimer's and other dementias. While science has failed to produce any effective dementia drugs, scientific studies prove we can do much by practicing healthy habits to slow or reduce our dementia risk.

The Medical Profession Must Think Outside The Box

The hopeless circle of failed drug trials demands we think outside the box or, as neurologist David Perlmutter advocates, expand the box. He and other neurologists deserve credit for recognizing medicine is failing the dementia war and rocking the boat of conventional wisdom. I must not agree with every point "maverick" neurologists like David Perlmutter, Dale Bredesen, and Deepak Chopra make to respect them for turning conventional wisdom on its head.

Conventional wisdom is losing the Alzheimer's and dementia war!

Not Anti-doctors or Anti-drugs

I am not anti-doctors or anti-drugs and do not understand those who insist neither are needed. I revere competent doctors who practice and advocate the three cornerstones of health. I also recognize the polio vaccine and many other drugs as nothing short of miraculous.

But, my love for what is right about the medical profession will not silence me about what is wrong. And, pretending drugs are the answer to defeating Alzheimer's or dementia is a colossal failure.

You cannot "**do no harm**" and write prescription drugs at the volume of the average doctor.

Choose A Doctor with The Same Care As You Do A Spouse

Find a competent, dedicated, caring, experienced, informed, ethical doctor who listens and respects your opinion, and writes prescriptions as a LAST RESORT.

Without the right doctor, you are at the mercy of a profit-oriented health system that seldom puts the patient's interests first, second, or third.

Nothing I say or write in these books or elsewhere means you should not see a doctor, stop taking your medication, or otherwise undermine the medical profession's ability to diagnose and treat any medical symptoms you might experience.

Find a good doctor you trust with your life and ask him or her pointed questions concerning your health and any treatment they recommend.

Outside the Bubble

I challenge the medical profession where necessary, just as I criticize Congress and the United States government for their mistakes or shortcomings. My brief career as a Congressional staffer taught me how difficult it is to maintain one's focus inside the bubble.

Seeing the big picture is no less challenging inside the medical bubble motivated by profit.

Profiteers fund too many studies to promote their product or discredit somebody else's. Blatant self-interests taint studies and confuse the public. Such contradictory studies confuse and make it impossible for the average person to understand which studies to believe.

I respect ethical, competent, dedicated, and hardworking nurses, doctors, and other medical personnel. As much as I criticize what is wrong within the profession, I cannot praise the majority of medical professionals often enough. Getting quality medical care when we need it is one of life's greatest blessings.

Nor do I object to medical-related businesses making a reasonable profit in return for needed medical supplies and services.

Nor should any competent and ethical medical professionals object to anybody challenging medical incompetence and profiteers.

Trust Thy Doctor

The right doctor does not discriminate between physical and mental diseases, so hold back nothing if you or a loved one exhibits symptoms.

If you lack the right doctor, find the right one. Outside you and the daily habits you establish, nobody is more important than your doctor for your health. You must be able to tell him or

NORMAL PRESSURE HYDROCEPHALUS

her medical information you might be reluctant to tell your closest confidant in life.

Remember, doctors too often misdiagnose dementia. Once the symptoms of these deadly dementias set in, you need to see your doctor, provide them with all the information about your problem, and help the specialists reach the correct diagnosis.

Because no tests exist for most dementias, doctors order tests and go through a process of elimination until reaching a diagnosis based on the symptoms you report. The more information you provide, the better the chance of a quick and accurate diagnosis.

Adopt healthy lifestyle choices to prevent dementia when possible, but the next best option is to diagnose it early, to confront it head-on, and take steps to slow the disease. Once dementia hits, it's often possible to postpone the advanced stages. If you've seen a loved one inflicted with dementia, you understand how precious a year, a month, a week, or day is once the storm aims at you or a loved one.

Prolonging life in late-stage dementia without a cure amounts to cruel and unusual punishment, but patients, families, and doctors must do everything possible to extend quality of life while possible.

Make certain you have a doctor who believes in prevention and natural cures, but also remember you need their expertise concerning the best that modern medicine offers.

Be Your Nurse!

If you have a loved one, be each other's nurse. If not, be your nurse.

It's more important than ever for you to monitor your blood pressure and make notes of health issues as they arise. We don't go to the doctor every time we develop a symptom or don't feel well, but it's important to keep a medical journal. Write an outline of the problems you experience between visits.

Too often, we march into the physician's office and don't provide a full or accurate representation of our problem. For instance, if you track your blood pressure, you can furnish a pattern rather than a onetime reading. You can also perhaps attribute pikes in your blood pressure to stress taking place in your life.

You should also track other symptoms. Providing thorough information helps doctors eliminate multiple diseases with similar symptoms. When you document all or most of the symptoms that have led to the visit, you provide a competent doctor a clearer picture to develop a hypothesis. These previous unrelated symptoms might help your physician make more sense of what prompted the appointment.

Otherwise, your physician might order the wrong tests or prescribe the wrong drugs. For issues of the brain, you can't be shy or embarrassed about providing your physician with a full portrayal of your problems and symptoms.

Although still stigmatized in some circles, mental illnesses are just as real, and the sufferers are no more the blame, than physical disorders. While we must do everything in our power to avoid or slow mental or physical maladies, the last thing we need to do is embarrass those who are already suffering.

Two Dementia Series

The laborious task to document the primary dementias began as a fifty-page Alzheimer's overview. Two editions later, the 50-page Alzheimer's book turned into 400 pages.

One of the first lessons taught Alzheimer's is only one of the hundreds of diseases responsible for dementia. With inadequate testing, similar symptoms, and other handicaps, the medical community often misdiagnoses the other dementias for Alzheimer's.

My focus broadened from Alzheimer's to a dozen dementias. The only way to make any sense of Alzheimer's or dementia was to study all the primary dementias.

I worked with several neurologists and researchers over the next couple of years and hit every medical library I could hit in person or available online.

After an extensive review, I wrote the first book covering the 15 most prevalent dementia types, which provided the groundwork for two updated dementia series.

The associated *Dementia Types, Symptoms, Stages, & Risk Factors, series* expands the collection by adding amyotrophic lateral sclerosis (ALS), early-onset Alzheimer's disease, amyotrophic lateral sclerosis, corticobasal syndrome, and progressive supranuclear palsy.

JERRY BELLER HEALTH RESEARCH INSTITUTE

Two Dementia Series

Not counting mixed dementia, there are nineteen primary dementia types, which two groundbreaking series covers.

Dementia Types, Symptoms, Stages, & Risk Factors series

1. *Dementia with Lewy Bodies*
2. *Parkinson's Disease Dementia*
3. Corticobasal Syndrome
4. Typical Alzheimer's Disease
5. *Posterior Cortical Atrophy*
6. *Down Syndrome with Alzheimer's*
7. *Limbic-predominant Age-related TDP-43 Encephalopathy (LATE)*
8. Early-onset Alzheimer's
9. *Behavioral Variant Frontotemporal Dementia*
10. Progressive Supranuclear Palsy
11. *Nonfluent Primary Progressive Aphasia*
12. Logopenic Progressive Aphasia
13. *Cortical Vascular Dementia*
14. *Binswanger Disease*
15. *Normal Pressure Hydrocephalus*
16. *Huntington's Disease*
17. *Korsakoff Syndrome*
18. *Creutzfeldt-Jakob Disease*
19. Amyotrophic Lateral Sclerosis

*Not a dementia type, but a combination, mixed dementia is the 20th category important in dementia discussions.

Any disease leading to associated symptoms is a dementia type. The series breaks medical ground by covering the dementias responsible for over 99% of dementia cases.

Dementia Overview Series

The second series focuses on all the primary dementia types or breaks them down as groups.

2020 Dementia Overview Series

1. *Dementia Types, Symptoms, & Stages*
2. *Lewy Body/Parkinsonism Dementias*
3. *Vascular Dementia*
4. *Frontotemporal Dementia (FTD)*
5. *Alzheimer's Related Dementias*
6. *Prevent or Slow Dementia*

The Best Science in Everyday Language

The text in both series contains American, Australian, British, and other English. I write in American English, but the research comes from the best studies worldwide. Quotes from the UK, Australia, and other English-speaking countries depend on the local dialect. For integrity, I do not edit quotes.

The books include facts and science as they exist. As much as possible, we replace medical jargon with everyday language.

Having explained the series, let's discuss dementia.

I. DEMENTIA

In this section, we discuss dementia.

Dementia is not a disease but a medical condition. Hundreds of diseases and disorders lead to dementia, but percentage-wise, almost all dementia falls under 19 primary dementia categories.

This series is the first to cover all 19 primary dementia types.

In this chapter, we answer the following questions:

- What is dementia?
- What are the 19 primary dementias?
- How prevalent is dementia?
- Who is most likely to get dementia?
- What are the financial costs to individuals, the U.S., and worldwide?

Once we answer these questions and provide a dementia overview, we turn our attention to the subject matter for the rest of the book.

Let's begin by answering the question: What is dementia?

Chapter 1: WHAT IS DEMENTIA?

For centuries, when one got dementia, people described the person in terms like "gone mad," or "lost their mind," or "crazy," or another derogatory term that missed the mark.

While most dementia types attack cognitive skills and cause behavioral disorders, the person is no less a victim than a cancer patient.

Whereas cancer attacks cells and organs, dementia destroys brain neurons.

The brain is complex. One-hundred billion neurons use over 100 trillion synapses and about 100 neurotransmitters to send all the signals to other parts of the brain, organs, and parts throughout the body, allowing us to think, reason, walk, talk, breathe, and do all that makes us human.

When fed, protected, and healthy, neurons perform magic.

The different dementias attack the brain and destroy the communication network responsible for everything our body does. By attacking different parts of the brain, the dementia types cause different disorders.

Let's see how some of the most prestigious American and global medical organizations define Dementia.

Alzheimer's Association Definition

Let's begin with the Alzheimer's Association:

> *Dementia is an overall term for diseases and conditions characterized by a decline in memory, language, problem-solving, and other thinking skills that affect a person's ability to perform everyday activities. Memory loss is an example. Alzheimer's is the most common cause of dementia*[1].

Dementia is to Alzheimer's, dementia with Lewy bodies,

Parkinson's dementia, vascular and the other dementia types what Asia is to China, India, North Korea, South Korea, and the rest of Asia. Alzheimer's is the most prevalent dementia, but each type devastates, and most are death sentences.

Let's turn to the National Institute on Aging (NIH) and see how they define dementia.

National Institute on Aging (NIH)

The National Institute on Aging (NIH) funds many studies and provides researchers invaluable data. How do they define dementia?

> *Dementia is the loss of cognitive functioning – thinking, remembering, and reasoning – and behavioral abilities to such an extent that it interferes with a person's daily life and activities. These functions include memory, language skills, visual perception, problem-solving, self-management, and the ability to focus and pay attention. Some people with dementia cannot control their emotions, and their personalities may change. Dementia ranges in severity from the mildest stage, when it is just beginning to affect a person's functioning, to the most severe stage, when the person must depend completely on others for basic activities of living*[2].

One of the most important things a person and their loved ones can do when diagnosed with dementia; enjoy what quality time remains.

Early diagnosis, medication, and lifestyle changes can slow the disease and extend quality life. From the point of diagnosis, make the most of each good day or moment.

Let's see how the international community defines dementia.

Alzheimer's Society UK

The Alzheimer's Society is perhaps the UK's most

prestigious Alzheimer's organization. They define dementia:

> *The word 'dementia' describes a set of symptoms that may include memory loss and difficulties with thinking, problem-solving or language. These changes are often small to start with, but for someone with dementia they have become severe enough to affect daily life. A person with dementia may also experience changes in their mood or behaviour[3].*

Let's see how the World Health Organization (WHO) defines dementia.

World Health Organization (WHO)

The World Health Organization (WHO) works with global medical organizations and provides researchers a wealth of information. How does WHO define dementia?

> *Dementia is a syndrome – usually of a chronic or progressive nature – in which there is deterioration in cognitive function (i.e. the ability to process thought) beyond what might be expected from normal ageing. It affects memory, thinking, orientation, comprehension, calculation, learning capacity, language, and judgement. Consciousness is not affected. The impairment in cognitive function is commonly accompanied, and occasionally preceded, by deterioration in emotional control, social behaviour, or motivation[4].*

The four organizations provide similar definitions, each emphasizing different points, but none contradicting the others.

Each organization confirms dementia is a broad neurological disorder. Hundreds of pathologies such as Alzheimer's leads to dementia, but 19 primary types cause about 99% of dementia cases. Dementia attacks the brain and causes memory decline, behavior disorders, motor decline, language deterioration, and most types are incurable.

If doctors diagnose you with dementia, you must get past the shock. Time is moving against you, so make the most of it.

As the Alzheimer's Society points out, the symptoms are minor in the beginning. Get your affairs in order, enjoy loved ones, and take part in as many activities as you desire and are able. To some extent, this is your farewell tour. Take advantage!

The disease will stop you or a loved one later, so do not stop living your life in the early stages.

Let's next examine the 19 primary dementia types.

Chapter 2: WHAT ARE THE 19 PRIMARY DEMENTIAS?

Hundreds of medical conditions lead to dementia, but 19 causes up to 99% of cases.

Each dementia type is devastating, most are fatal, and the first symptoms to death is a challenging, heartbreaking, soul-crushing experience. Dementia robs the personalities and functionality of marvelous people a little at a time until they no longer resemble the person they've always been.

19 Dementia Types

This chapter divides the 19 primary dementias into six categories. The first group includes dementias related to Lewy body or Parkinsonism dementia. The second consists of Alzheimer's-related dementia. In the third, we focus on primary progressive aphasia dementias. The fourth contains vascular dementias. The fifth category encompasses the remaining dementias and is called *other dementias*.

Lewy Body/Parkinsonism Related Dementias

1. *Dementia with Lewy Bodies*
2. *Parkinson's Disease Dementia*
3. Corticobasal Syndrome

Alzheimer's Related Dementias

4. Typical Alzheimer's Disease
5. Posterior Cortical Atrophy
6. Down Syndrome with Alzheimer's
7. Limbic-predominant Age-related TDP-43 Encephalopathy (LATE)
8. Early-onset Alzheimer's

Frontotemporal Lobar Degeneration Related Dementias

9. *Behavioral Variant Frontotemporal Dementia*
10. Progressive Supranuclear Palsy

Primary Progressive Aphasia Related Dementias

11. *Nonfluent Primary Progressive Aphasia (nfvPPA)*
12. Logopenic Progressive Aphasia (LPA)

Vascular Dementia

13. *Cortical Vascular Dementia*
14. *Binswanger Disease*

Other Dementias

15. *Normal Pressure Hydrocephalus*
16. *Huntington's Disease*
17. *Korsakoff Syndrome*
18. *Creutzfeldt-Jakob Disease*
19. Amyotrophic Lateral Sclerosis

Chapter 3: WHO IS MOST LIKELY TO GET DEMENTIA?

In this chapter, we explore who is most likely to get dementia. Most know people with dementia are old, but some people are born with dementia, others get it as infants, and the disease attacks people in every age group.

There are risk factors that affect everybody. Examples include a poor diet, lack of exercise, diabetes, obesity, high blood pressure, and factors under and beyond our control.

In this chapter, we focus on risk factors affecting specific groups of people who suffer higher rates.

The research pointed to age, race, and sex, where dementia seems to discriminate. Let's review the science for each.

Age

Age is the obvious risk factor. We know because of science and our observations.

So associated with the elderly, many believe dementia only strikes older people. However, dementia strikes all ages and demographics, including newborns and infants.

According to Stanford University Medical School, "The risk of Alzheimer's disease, vascular dementia, and several other dementias goes up significantly with advancing age[5]."

None of us enjoy aging. We must work harder and harder to slow aging, and no matter how well we do, none of us will make it much past 100 years. The better we take care of ourselves, the higher chance we have of living a quality life into our eighties or nineties.

Remember, aging does not destroy our cognitive abilities. Bad habits do! I stress this point because each of us can slow the aging process through healthy habits.

As people age, however, our dementia risks increase.

A Journal of Neurology, Neurosurgery, & Psychiatry study concluded[6]:

> *In the age group 65–69 years, there are more than two new cases per 1000 persons every year. This number increases almost exponentially with increasing age, until over the age of 90 years, out of 1000 persons, 70 new cases of dementia can be expected every year.*

As we stress in our book on prevention, there is actual age and real age. We determine one's actual age by the day and year born, whereas weight, blood pressure, blood sugar, cholesterol, diet, how often you work out, and several other important factors govern our real age.

Unless genes or an accident prevents us, our real age should be lower than our actual age. Those who practice bad habits, however, raise their real age ten years or more than their actual age.

When our real age is lower than our actual age, we lower our risks for dementia and other diseases. When our real age is higher than our actual age, we increase risks for dementia, heart disease, cancer, and all major diseases.

Let's next review if race plays a role in dementia.

Race

African Americans and blacks in western countries suffer more than their share of racism.

The United States has abused too many citizens since its creation, but none more than Native Americans and African Americans.

But, does dementia also discriminate against them?

According to AARP, African Americans are 64% more likely to get dementia than non-Hispanic whites[7].

Kaiser Permanente Study

Researchers in another study examined data from 274,000 Kaiser Permanente patients over 14 years. They found the highest rate of dementia for African Americans and Native Americans[8].

Dementia Risk Per 1,000 People

- 27 African Americans
- 22 Native Americans
- 20 Latinos and Pacific Islanders
- 19 White Americans
- 15 Asian-Americans

Does dementia love Asian and European-Americans and hate African and Native-Americans?

Dementia is as evil as the worst bigot, but dementia is not a bigot.

African Americans experience higher rates of diabetes. African Americans and Native Americans suffer a higher level of stress, poverty, and disenfranchisement. Both cultures also struggle with their people's history in European-America and endure a greater level of bigotry and more obstacles to succeeding in modern America.

On the flip side, Asian Americans and whites have lower obesity and diabetes rates, eat a more balanced diet, faceless bigotry, are more affluent, educated, and successful in modern America.

We need more studies to confirm the exact causes of higher dementia incidence in the African and Native American populations. Higher stress and diabetes in their communities are prime suspects.

Jennifer Manly, Columbia University, Taub Institute for Research on Alzheimer's disease, and Aging Brain spoke to Reuters about the inequities.

> *There are huge disparities in dementia that are confronting this nation and this will translate into an enormous burden on families if we don't address this. We need to prioritize research that uncovers the reasons for these disparities and more research should include racially and ethnically diverse people[9].*

Are African British at a greater risk for Dementia?

In the United Kingdom, black women are 25% more likely than white women, and black men 28% more likely than white men to get dementia[10].

Reluctance to Take Part in Dementia Studies

African Americans and Native Americans are also less trustful of studies. Too often in the past, a bigoted establishment treated African Americans and Native Americans like lab rats.

The awful past makes the average African American reluctant to take part in studies that might help us figure out how to lower the rates.

Native Americans are also distrustful of the United States government and the "white man's studies," as one group from the Cherokee Reservation in North Carolina told me.

I understand both ethnic groups' skepticism. As somebody with ancestors who died and survived the Trail of Tears, and who married a black woman (30+ years), nobody must convince me of the tainted American history. I have read about the past and viewed enough with my own eyes to know the sins of America's past, either haunt or still torment today.

But, the Studies are Necessary!

I call on African Americans and Native Americans to take part in dementia studies. The studies today have greater safeguards than the past and face much more scrutiny.

Dementia is a death sentence!

Worse than the average killer, never content to kill and move on, dementia is a sadist. Dementia destroys the mind and body, little by little, robbing one's personality, dignity, mind, body, and everything that makes a person unique.

If African Americans and Native Americans refuse to participate in dementia studies, fatal neurological disorders will continue to strike them worse than other ethnic groups.

Please consider two facts.

If you do not have dementia, researchers do not subject you to drug trials but accumulate data to determine which habits increase and decrease one's risks.

If doctors diagnose you with dementia, trials represent your last best chance to win what is otherwise a losing battle.

What Role does Poverty Play?

Although not listed as a dementia risk factor, poverty increases one's risk for almost every significant disease. Those at the bottom must worry where the next meal is coming, if somebody might mug (or kill) them when leaving the house, and a laundry list of stress the average citizen seems oblivious.

Beller Health calls for more research to determine if Native American, African American, and African British citizens have higher dementia rates as a general population, or if poverty drives these numbers. We need to know whether the number also applies to middle-and upper-class African Americans and Native Americans who eat healthily, exercise, do not abuse alcohol, avoid tobacco, and do not abuse prescription or illicit drugs.

Native American, African American, and African British citizens suffer a higher percentage of poverty than other demographics in the US and UK.

Rather than race, such factors as poverty, bigotry, and lack of opportunities might drive these numbers.

I reached out to several organizations, including the VA, to conduct a large-scale study to determine what role poverty plays in dementia. Most organizations greeted my request with enthusiasm, and I hope one or more soon back the study.

All we know for certain is poverty in the industrial world causes a much greater level of stress and other hardships than the rest of the population. WHO reported that about 60% of dementia cases occur in the poorest half of countries[11].

Age and ethnicity are dementia risk factors. What about sex?

Sex

Dementia strikes older people, African Americans, Native Americans, and African British in greater numbers than the rest of the population. Does one's gender increase or decrease one's odds?

How Many Women have Dementia?

According to the Alzheimer's Association, women represent two-thirds of people living with Alzheimer's, and 13 million women suffer dementia or are caring for somebody who does[12].

Of the 820,000 people living with dementia in the UK, females account for 61 percent[13].

Of the 50 million people living with dementia worldwide[14], women represent 65 percent[15].

Key points:

- Women represent two-thirds of Alzheimer's cases.
- Females account for 65% of dementia cases.

Is dementia just another woman-hating predator?

Does Alzheimer's & Most Dementia Strike Women in Greater Numbers?

While the two key numbers suggest dementia is a rampaging woman-abusing murderer, the answer is not so simple.

While women represent two-thirds of Alzheimer's cases and 65% of dementia cases, there are 19 primary dementia types.

Some dementias attack men in greater numbers and much harder than females. The dementias we know attack men in greater ratios include[16]:

- Parkinson's dementia (Lewy body dementia)
- Dementia with Lewy bodies (Lewy body dementia)
- Post-Stroke dementia (Vascular dementia)
- Multi-infarct dementia (Vascular dementia)
- Binswanger Disease(Vascular dementia)
- Normal pressure hydrocephalus
- Behavioral variant frontotemporal dementia
- Primary Progressive Aphasia (Frontotemporal dementia)
- Chronic traumatic encephalopathy
- HIV-related cognitive impairment
- Amyotrophic lateral sclerosis

From the data about the 19 primary dementias, at least eleven attack men in greater numbers. Data is not available for Creutzfeldt-Jakob disease, Wernicke-Korsakoff Syndrome, LATE, and Down syndrome with Alzheimer's disease. The remaining dementias strike both genders in similar numbers.

When the authorities release more information, we will update this section.

If a minimum of 11 of 19 dementia types strike men in greater numbers than women, how can 68% of people living with dementia be women?

Alzheimer's accounts for 60-80% of dementia, and two-thirds of people with Alzheimer's are women.

When we say dementia attacks, women, 65% to 35% men, we distort the picture. I call on the medical community to provide greater clarity. More precise, we should warn women to represent two-thirds of total Alzheimer's cases, but stress a minimum of 11 of 19 dementia types strike men in greater numbers.

Treating dementia and Alzheimer's as interchangeable terms is misleading. There are 19 primary dementias and 11 or more attack men in greater numbers. If we exclude Alzheimer's and focus on the other 18 primary dementia types, they attack men by far greater percentages.

With that stipulation, let's explore why Alzheimer's and some dementias attack women more than men.

Why Does Alzheimer's & Dementia Strike Women in Greater Numbers Than Men?

In part, unique burdens & responsibilities explain the disparity.

Women still fight today for equality. Like Native Americans, African Americans, and African British, the average woman carries burdens; the average man is clueless.

To be a woman, one fights for equality from birth in a "man's world," as the song and tradition attest. Among things unique to women:

- Menstrual cycles (ranging from mild to horrendous)
- Childbirth
- Menopause

Being a guy is also difficult, but there's no denying women are born with unique responsibilities and burdens.

As an aunt once retorted, if they live long enough, every woman suffers menstrual cycles until menopause "tortures it out."

Women Live Longer

Women outlive men in the United States and worldwide.

Worldwide, the average man lives to age 69.8, while the average woman lives 74.2 years[17]. These are the average numbers, so they fluctuate from region to region and country to country.

Let's see how these numbers compare to the United States.

American Comparisons

The CDC reports the average American male lives 76 years, compared to the average American woman who lives 81 years[18].

Why Do Women Live Longer Than Men?

Although women live longer, this might result because more men abuse alcohol, tobacco, and drugs, get less sleep, work in more hazardous jobs, suffer greater casualties in war, and take unnecessary risks.

The lead author of a study published in the *British Medical Journal*, Australian neuropsychiatrist Richard Cibulskis, confirmed some of my suspicions.

> *Men are much more likely to die from preventable and treatable non-communicable diseases, such as {ischemic} heart disease and lung cancer, and road traffic accidents*[19].

Global population expert, Dr. Perminder Sachdev, confirmed my other suspicions in an interview with *Time*.

"Men are more likely to smoke, drink excessively and be overweight," Sachdev said. "They are also less likely to seek medical help early, and, if diagnosed with a disease, they are more likely to be non-adherent to treatment." Sachdev also pointed out, "men are more likely to take life-threatening risks and to die in car accidents, brawls or gunfights[20]."

Although nature perhaps installed a natural order to preserve the female population, men's reckless nature might account for the five years difference in life expectancy between the genders.

It will interest to see if the numbers change as more women become more like men. Women are assuming greater roles in war, law enforcement, and other areas where even men with healthy habits have fallen. As the societal lines between men and women blur, the difference in life expectancy should fall.

In all honorable fields of life, women should go for it. Never has there been a better time to prove the equality of the sexes.

As far as men's bad habits, my hope is women continue to show better judgment and exercise greater restraint. Women will never prove their equality by emulating men's worse habits or trying to outdo us in the stupid department.

The best men and women rise on similar foundations. However, the worst men and women also share a foundation. My hope for humans getting our act together soon hinges on the average woman being better than the average man.

Love yourselves for your unique feminine qualities. Be equal, but please do not confuse out-drinking, out-smoking, out-drugging, acting more reckless, and stupid than men with being equal. We need fewer men like that, not more women!

Chapter 4: DEMENTIA COSTS & PREVALENCE

In this chapter, we review dementia prevalence and costs to governments, the world, caregivers, and patients.

How Many People Worldwide Suffer Dementia?

According to the World Health Organization (WHO), over 50 million people suffer dementia worldwide, with 10 million new cases each year[21].

How Many Americans Have Dementia?

In the United States, 5.8 million Americans live with dementia[22], with Alzheimer's representing 70% of cases.

Let's check the UK dementia numbers.

How Many People In The UK Have Dementia?

According to the Alzheimer's Society, 850,000 people in the UK live with dementia[23].

Alzheimer's Society reports that about 70% of those living in UK care homes suffer dementia.

The numbers show Americans, British, and global citizens suffering high rates of dementia. Let's see which countries' dementia strikes the hardest.

Which Countries Have The Highest Dementia Rate?

Per World Atlas, the following ten countries suffer the highest dementia rate of deaths per 100,000 people[24]:

1. Finland
2. USA
3. Canada
4. Iceland
5. Sweden
6. Switzerland
7. Norway
8. Denmark
9. The Netherlands
10. Belgium

As we review the list, per population, dementia strikes Americans in greater numbers than any country but Finland.

Why?

There are several explanations:

- Over two-thirds of Americans are obese or overweight.
- The other countries on the list also suffer higher obesity levels than most countries not on the list.
- Because of weight issues, the countries in question suffer high rates of diabetes and high blood pressure, both dementia risk factors.
- Americans consume more prescription drugs than people worldwide. While there is no data to confirm, I suspect the other countries on the list also have greater access and use more prescription drugs than poorer countries.
- They load the western diet with salt, sugar, and

white processed flours.
- The average person in western countries lives longer than those in poorer nations.
- We will add other factors once data becomes available.
- People live longer in these countries than most not on the list (the older one lives, the greater the dementia risk)

Another explanation is more misdiagnosis and no-diagnosis in poorer countries around the world. Obesity and other risk factors are also less of a problem in developing countries.

I recommend global researchers compare the ten countries on this list. By viewing the similarities between the ten, we might better pinpoint the cause for Alzheimer's and the other dementias.

If we can figure out what the citizens from the ten nations are doing wrong, we can find the cause and means of preventing dementia. While I pointed to some of the most obvious risk factors, the most important common risk factor from the ten nations might be something unexpected.

Let's now examine dementia costs.

Dementia Costs

In this chapter, we analyze dementia costs. We examine the United States and global costs, then provide estimated costs per family.

What Does Dementia Cost the United States?

More than the entire economies of Finland and 166 other countries, dementia costs the United States $277 billion per year.

What Does Dementia Cost Worldwide?

Getting credible global numbers proves difficult, if not impossible, in any medical research. Often, the best source is the World Health Organization (WHO). They collect data from around the world and are an essential source for medical researchers.

Getting accurate dementia numbers in richer countries is difficult. In the United States and the UK, black people hesitate to take part in dementia studies or to seek medical attention for symptoms.

In richer countries, there are still too many misdiagnoses.

Thus, if we cannot get ironclad numbers in the United States, the United Kingdom, and the industrial nations, the task proves even more difficult for developing countries.

If the United States and the United Kingdom have difficulty convincing black citizens to seek medical attention for dementia symptoms, the third world faces even greater obstacles.

In the third world, most areas do well to offer their citizens basic medical care. With no urine or blood test, many regions lack resources for CAT scans, MRIs, and other expensive imaging equipment to make a diagnosis.

Without urine or blood tests, diagnosing dementia costs more than low-income people with inadequate or no insurance can afford in the richest countries.

In the United States and industrial nations, doctors often misdiagnose the other 19 primary dementias for Alzheimer's or each other.

Expecting doctors in many third world nations to diagnose dementia with inferior or no equipment is to expect miracles. If it overwhelms medical professionals in the wealthier nations, we often expect third world doctors to perform miracles. What amazes is they often do!

However, no matter how good a job the average third world doctor does treating typical medical conditions, even if trained, it does not equip them to diagnose dementia early, if at all. My comments are not criticism.

The average doctor's job is not to diagnose or treat dementia, but they must recognize symptoms and refer the patient to neurologists. Primary care physicians are the first line of defense.

North, south, east, west, dementia overwhelms the medical community.

Having discussed the limitations, let's examine the data. While the numbers are ballpark figures, landing in the park is the keystone to estimation. In most cases, the real numbers are much higher.

According to the *World Alzheimer's Report,* global dementia costs a minimum of $1 trillion per year, and experts predict it will reach $2 trillion by 2030 if we find no cure[25].

Authorities should release new numbers over the next year, and we will update this section.

The *Alzheimer's Report* global cost estimations do not include informal care costs; another reason we consider the estimates conservative.

The Alzheimer's Report concluded:

> *Direct medical care costs account for roughly 20% of global dementia costs, while direct social sector costs and informal care costs each account for roughly 40%. The relative contribution of informal care is greatest in the African regions and lowest in North America, Western Europe and some South American regions, while the reverse is true for social sector costs.*

Whatever the real up-to-date costs, we must take action to reduce the burden on individuals and nations. If we do not invest in independent research to develop an effective urine or blood test, cure, and vaccine for each dementia type, the costs will smother economies throughout the world. The costs will cripple developing countries and destabilize the wealthiest.

We have no choice but to invest more in dementia research. No matter which country you live, your economy, security, and the health of your nation rides on us finding a cure or vaccine.

As a scientist, I find it disturbing climate change and independent dementia research are not major priorities. Most governments, businesses, and individuals who can afford to fund dementia remain MIA in the war against dementia.

Before we conclude this section, let's examine the dementia statistics side-by-side in the table below.

DEMENTIA STATISTICS

This table focuses on the number of people with dementia and the number of deaths per 100,000 among the nations chosen for comparison.

NATION	# OF PEOPLE WITH DEMENTIA	DEMENTIA DEATHS PER 100,000 PEOPLE	TOTAL COSTS (US DOLLARS)
Australia	447,115	29.61	$15 billion
Brazil	1 million +	10.71	$16.45 billion
Canadian	747,000	37.30	$10.4 billion
China	16.93 million	19.87	$69 billion
France	1.2 million	30.84	$37.91 billion
Germany	1.5 million	16.99	$57.57 billion
India	4 million	14.57	$28.38 billion
Italy	1.4 million	19.81	$29.96 billion
Japan	4.6 million	7.22	$14.8 billion
Mexico	800,000	3.62	Not available
Spain	800.000+	29.23	$19.98 million
Netherlands	280,000	39.37	$4.44 million
United States	5.8 million	44.41	$290 billion
United Kingdom	850,000	49.18	$26.3 billion

Sources: World Health Rankings[26], Alzheimer's Europe[27], NATSIM[28], Alzheimer's Society[29], Brain Test[30]

Other sources cited in the chapter.

The table comes from my book 2020 Dementia Overview, which covers cost and prevalence among comparative nations in greater detail.

Let's next discuss the dementia costs for caregivers.

What Does Dementia Cost Volunteer Caregivers?

Although 41% make less than $50,000, American voluntary caregivers devote a minimum of 18.4 billion hours per year to dementia patients.

Worth $232 billion per year, we underrate the voluntary caregiving heroes in our fight against dementia. This total does not include lost wages for the voluntary caregiver.

According to the Northwestern Mutual C.A.R.E. Study, 67% of voluntary caregivers must cut their living to help pay for the patient's medical care, and 57% end up experiencing financial problems[31].

Adding to the costs of voluntary caregivers, they often end up sick themselves. Caring for loved ones with dementia bankrupts many.

In the early stages, the loved one can still perform most of their daily tasks but will require 24/7 care once the symptoms advance.

Imagine putting your life on hold for years to care, bathe, feed, protect, and take such a heavy load on your shoulders.

Millions of dementia families face the dilemma where the husband and wife both must work in most families to get by. You work as a couple to build stability in your own family, and then, boom, doctors diagnose one of you with dementia.

What Does Dementia Cost Dementia Patients?

When we say patient, past a certain stage in the disease, we refer to family or loved ones. A person who cannot perform daily tasks cannot manage finances, even if they have any left.

Too often, the costs drive entire families into bankruptcy because of dementia costs for a member.

Authorities estimate the average cost per dementia patient is $341,840, with families expected to cover 70 percent.

The costs devastate the average family in the industrial nations.

How are they supposed to afford it in developing countries where the average citizen makes less than one-thousand American dollars per year?

Dementia Recap

Although your dementia research has just begun, you now have a decent overview of Dementia.

In Chapter One, we explored dementia. We turned to several top dementia or medical organizations and compared their definitions.

Chapter two explained Alzheimer's is to dementia what China is to Asia. We listed the 19 dementias. They include:

1. Dementia with Lewy Bodies
2. Parkinson's Disease Dementia
3. Corticobasal Syndrome
4. Typical Alzheimer's Disease
5. Posterior Cortical Atrophy
6. Down Syndrome with Alzheimer's
7. Limbic-predominant Age-related TDP-43 Encephalopathy (LATE)
8. Early-onset Alzheimer's
9. Behavioral Variant Frontotemporal Dementia
10. Progressive Supranuclear Palsy
11. Nonfluent Primary Progressive Aphasia
12. Logopenic Progressive Aphasia
13. Cortical Vascular Dementia
14. Binswanger Disease
15. Normal Pressure Hydrocephalus
16. Huntington's Disease
17. Korsakoff Syndrome
18. Creutzfeldt-Jakob Disease
19. Amyotrophic Lateral Sclerosis

Although most the dementia types share similar symptoms, enough to cause misdiagnosis, each has its unique pathology and symptoms.

In chapter three, we explored dementia prevalence in the United States, the UK, and worldwide.

Chapter four examined who is most likely to get dementia. We found Native Americans (those who greeted the first Europeans), and black citizens in the United States and the UK are more likely to get dementia than their white or Asian counterparts.

We also explored the women to men ratio. Women represent two-thirds of Alzheimer's and over sixty percent of dementia cases. We pointed out the Alzheimer's figure skews the dementia numbers because men are more likely to get a minimum of 11 of the 19 primary dementia types.

Chapter four explored the US, UK, global, patient, family, and voluntary caregivers' dementia costs. The staggering numbers are almost as frightening as the medical disorder itself.

We borrowed the following table from *2020 Dementia Overview.*

Dementia Costs & Prevalence

NATION	# OF PEOPLE WITH DEMENTIA	DEMENTIA DEATHS PER 100,000 PEOPLE	TOTAL COSTS (US DOLLARS)
Australia	447,115	29.61	$15 billion
Brazil	1 million +	10.71	$16.45 billion
Canadian	747,000	37.30	$10.4 billion
China	16.93 million	19.87	$69 billion
France	1.2 million	30.84	$37.91 billion
Germany	1.5 million	16.99	$57.57 billion
India	4 million	14.57	$28.38 billion
Italy	1.4 million	19.81	$29.96 billion
Japan	4.6 million	7.22	$14.8 billion
Mexico	800,000	3.62	Not available
Spain	800.000+	29.23	$19.98 million
Netherlands	280,000	39.37	$4.44 million
United States	5.8 million	44.41	$290 billion
United Kingdom	850,000	49.18	$26.3 billion

Sources: World Health Rankings[32], Alzheimer's Europe[33], NATSIM[34], Alzheimer's Society[35], Brain Test[36]

The table comes from 2020 Dementia Overview, which covers cost and prevalence among comparative nations in greater detail.

After reviewing the conservative numbers, and factoring in an aging population, we concluded we must find a cure before it bankrupts millions of families and cripples nations.

Having explained the series and introduced dementia, let's discuss normal pressure hydrocephalus.

II. NORMAL PRESSURE HYDROCEPHALUS

This section shifts the focus to this book's specific topic, normal pressure hydrocephalus.

Chapter 5: WHAT IS HYDROCEPHALUS?

Let's begin our discussion by defining the word hydrocephalus. *Hydro*[37] means water and *cephalus*[38] imply head.

The American Association of Neurological Surgeons describes hydrocephalus:

> Hydrocephalus is a condition in which excess cerebrospinal fluid (CSF) builds up within the ventricles (fluid-containing cavities) of the brain and may increase pressure within the head. Although hydrocephalus is often described as "water on the brain," the "water" is actually CSF, a clear fluid surrounding the brain and spinal cord. CSF has three crucial functions: 1) it acts as a "shock absorber" for the brain and spinal cord; 2) it acts as a vehicle for delivering nutrients to the brain and removing waste; and 3) it flows between the cranium and spine to regulate changes in pressure within the brain[39].

Understanding hydrocephalus requires a basic knowledge of the brain, spinal cord, ventricles, and cerebrospinal fluid.

Let's view a hydrocephalus brain and see what causes the problem.

Hydrocephalus Brain

Let's look at the brain with hydrocephalus.

Hydrocephalus

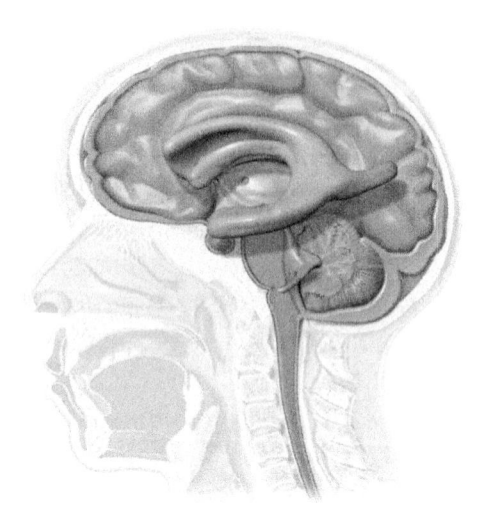

As you see in the image, too much cerebrospinal fluid bulges and damages the brain and spinal cord, causing hydrocephalus.

Primary Hydrocephalus Types

The two primary hydrocephalus types are communicating hydrocephalus and noncommunicating hydrocephalus, but there are five other classifications:

- Normal pressure hydrocephalus
- Hydrocephalus ex-vacuo
- Acquired hydrocephalus
- Congenital hydrocephalus
- Compensated hydrocephalus

Let's discuss communicating and noncommunicating hydrocephalus; then, we will discuss the other classifications.

Communicating Hydrocephalus

Our primary focus is communicating hydrocephalus (CH), or, more specifically, one of CH's subtypes, normal pressure hydrocephalus.

Medscape describes communicating hydrocephalus:

> *Communicating hydrocephalus occurs when full communication occurs between the ventricles and subarachnoid space. It is caused by overproduction of CSF (rarely), defective absorption of CSF (most often, includes conditions such as intracranial hemorrhage or meningitis resulting in damage to the arachnoid granulations, where CSF is reabsorbed), or venous drainage insufficiency (occasionally)*[40].

The primary communicating subtype is normal pressure hydrocephalus (NPHP), an accurate name despite everybody's first reaction: *What's normal about hydrocephalus?*

Communicating Normal Pressure Hydrocephalus

Medical authorities refer to hydrocephalus as communicating when cerebrospinal fluid flows uninterrupted through the brain's subarachnoid space and the ventricular system.

Although rarer than Alzheimer's, Lewy body dementia, vascular dementia, and frontotemporal dementia, normal pressure hydrocephalus is yet another death-dealing disease. National Institute of Neurological Disorders and Stroke describe normal pressure hydrocephalus as one of the most mysterious dementias[41]:

> *Normal pressure hydrocephalus (NPH) is an abnormal buildup of cerebrospinal fluid (CSF) in the brain's ventricles, or cavities. It occurs if the normal flow of CSF throughout the brain and spinal cord is blocked in some way. This causes the ventricles to enlarge, putting pressure on the*

brain. Normal pressure hydrocephalus can occur in people of any age, but it is most common in the elderly. It may result from a subarachnoid hemorrhage, head trauma, infection, tumor, or complications of surgery. However, many people develop NPH even when none of these factors are present. In these cases the cause of the disorder is unknown.

Since normal pressure hydrocephalus is a less prevalent form of dementia, it's likely to be years before we figure out these "unknown" causes.

Diagnosing normal pressure hydrocephalus is difficult because some symptoms overlap with Alzheimer's and other dementias. As every normal pressure hydrocephalus organization, researcher, or doctor attests, we need more funding for vital research.

We need to know the exact cause or causes to help develop urine or blood tests, vaccines, and cures.

Noncommunicating Obstructive Hydrocephalus

Unlike communicating, which happens between the ventricles and the subarachnoid space, noncommunicating or obstructive hydrocephalus occurs in the ventricle-connecting passages. Also known as obstructive hydrocephalus, noncommunicating hydrocephalus often takes place between the third and fourth ventricles in the Sylvius's aqueduct narrowing[42].

Doctors refer to hydrocephalus as non-communicating when a tumor or something blocks or inhibits cerebrospinal fluid in the ventricular system.

Other Hydrocephalus Classifications

There are four other hydrocephalus forms worth noting.

Hydrocephalus Ex-vacuo

This type results from traumatic brain injuries, stroke, or dementia such as Alzheimer's. Hydrocephalus ex-vacuo often shrinks brain tissue.

Acquired Hydrocephalus

Acquired normal pressure hydrocephalus occurs at or after birth.

Congenital Hydrocephalus

Babies with congenital normal pressure hydrocephalus are born with the disease.

Compensated Hydrocephalus

Compensated hydrocephalus is present at birth or in early childhood, but lingers, showing no symptoms into adulthood.

How Many People have Normal Pressure Hydrocephalus?

According to the Hydrocephalus Association, over 700,000 Americans suffer normal pressure hydrocephalus, but doctors often misdiagnose the symptoms as Parkinson's disease or Alzheimer's disease[43].

The number might be much higher.

According to the Cleveland Clinic[44], "as many as 10 percent of people with dementia attributed to other disorders may actually have NPH {normal pressure hydrocephalus)."

Misdiagnosis

I blame misdiagnoses on four factors.

One, over 100 diseases are leading to dementia, and most share some symptoms. Two, with no blood or urine test for most, one cannot confirm the diagnosis for many dementias until postmortem during an autopsy. Three, there is not enough money to fund all the needed Alzheimer's studies, much less the lesser-known dementias, meaning we've barely broken the research surface for some. Four, diagnosing dementia is expensive and requires running imaging and other tests often not covered by insurance. Five, undertraining, or incompetence causes some misdiagnosis, with undertraining probably most serious.

Who gets Normal Pressure Hydrocephalus?

Normal pressure hydrocephalus strikes most people over sixty[45] but attacks people all ages, including newborns.

How Many Babies are Born with Normal Pressure Hydrocephalus?

Two of 1,000 babies are born with normal pressure hydrocephalus[46].

Is there a Cure for Normal Pressure Hydrocephalus?

Most dementias are incurable, but—if diagnosed early enough—the medical profession might reverse normal pressure hydrocephalus[47].

What are the Medical Costs for Normal Pressure Hydrocephalus?

Normal pressure hydrocephalus medical costs surpass $2 billion per year[48].

What causes Normal Pressure Hydrocephalus (NPH)?

What Causes Normal Pressure Hydrocephalus?

Researchers uncovered two pathways to normal pressure hydrocephalus:

1. Primary (idiopathic)
2. Secondary

Primary Normal Pressure Hydrocephalus

If I hate the name normal pressure hydrocephalus, which I do, I profoundly dislike when we do not know the exact causes of neurological disorders. Normal Pressure Hydrocephalus cause remains unknown.

Secondary Normal Pressure Hydrocephalus

Tumors, subarachnoid hemorrhages, and head injuries are the primary causes of this version[49].

III. NORMAL PRESSURE HYDROCEPHALUS SYMPTOMS

Chapter 6: NORMAL PRESSURE HYDROCEPHALUS SYMPTOMS (NPH)

Normal pressure hydrocephalus lacks the stages established for Alzheimer's and most dementias because it lags in research. Also, unlike other dementias, normal pressure hydrocephalus is often reversible. Therefore, it does not follow typical dementia stages.

We know the symptoms and, if untreated, grow more severe. Untreated or maltreated, normal pressure hydrocephalus causes premature death like most dementias.

As somebody who studies all the primary dementias, I enjoy researching normal pressure hydrocephalus. Not only do I find medical research fascinating, but there are positive outcomes.

If diagnosed and treated early, neurologists often reverse normal pressure hydrocephalus. Like anybody else, I love happy endings.

Let's discuss the most common normal pressure hydrocephalus symptoms.

What Are Symptoms Of Normal Pressure Hydrocephalus (NPH)?

Let's breakdown symptoms for primary and secondary NPH. This form leads to gait problems, urinary incontinence, and dementia[50].

The symptoms and progression differ from patient-to-patient, but below are common.

- Attention-deficit[51]
- Bradyphrenia[52] (rigidity, weakness, tremors)
- Freezing (feeling as if one's feet stick to the floor)
- Impaired thinking skills[53]
- Inability to control the bladder (incontinence)[54]
- Irritability[55]
- Memory loss[56]
- Shuffled gait
- Walking difficulty[57]
- Injury from fall[58]

The gait and balance bladder issues are more pronounced in the beginning than cognitive issues[59].

Normal pressure hydrocephalus requires more studies, but this is one form of dementia that neurosurgeons can reduce through surgery if caught soon enough[60]. Unless examined by a neurosurgeon, doctors often misdiagnose normal pressure hydrocephalus.

Children and adults experience different normal pressure hydrocephalus. Because their fibrous joints connecting bones in the skull are unclosed, children can better adapt to cerebrospinal fluid buildup than adults.

Most Obvious Normal Pressure Hydrocephalus Symptoms for Children

While children better adapt to the cerebrospinal fluid buildup, their heads grow unusually large.

Other Normal Pressure Hydrocephalus Symptoms for Children

- Head soft spot bulges
- Skullbone gaps (split sutures)
- Irritability
- Seizures
- Sleepy
- Sun setting (Downward eyes)
- Swollen veins
- Vomiting

Normal Pressure Hydrocephalus Symptoms for Older Children & Adults

As we age, the more our heads and brains set, so the initial symptoms are more severe for older children and adults.

Most older children and adults with normal pressure hydrocephalus first suffer headaches.

Cerebrospinal fluid buildup puts pressure on the brain.

Other Normal Pressure Hydrocephalus Symptoms for Older Children & Adults

While they vary from one person to the next, symptoms for adults and older children include a variety of physical, cognitive, and urinary issues.

- Blurred vision
- Depression
- Double vision
- Cognitive decline
- Drowsy
- Gait decline
- Impaired coordination
- Irritable
- Lethargic
- Memory loss
- Nausea
- Poor balance
- Sun setting
- Urinary incontinence
- Vomiting

Parkinson's disease and Creutzfeldt-Jakob share a long list of symptoms, explaining why doctors often misdiagnose normal pressure hydrocephalus.

Symptoms Sources: American Association of Neurological Surgeons[61], Joseph H. Piatt Jr., MD[62], Child Neurology Foundation[63], Harvard Medical School[64], National Organization of Rare Disorders[65] (NORD), Johns Hopkins Medicine[66], National Health Service[67] (NHS),

III. NORMAL PRESSURE HYDROCEPHALUS STAGES

Now that we've listed the symptoms, let's cover the stages for normal pressure hydrocephalus.

Chapter 7: NORMAL PRESSURE HYDROCEPHALUS (NPH) STAGES

Normal-pressure hydrocephalus (NPH) lacks the stages established for Alzheimer's. NPH severity depends on initial damage and how soon one sees a doctor.

Also, unlike other dementias, normal pressure hydrocephalus is often reversible.

The symptoms, if untreated, grow more severe. Untreated or maltreated, normal pressure hydrocephalus causes premature death like most dementias.

Earliest Symptoms

In the beginning, one often suffers gait disruption, featuring wide, shuffled, slow, short steps. Depending on the initial brain damage, the gait ranges from mild to a full walking and standing disability[68].

If treated, neurosurgeons often can improve or reverse the condition. If untreated, the symptoms grow progressively worse.

Next Symptoms

Not far behind the gait problems, many develop cognitive or psychological symptoms[69].

Whether one experiences cognitive issues, most develop bladder control problems not long after the initial gait symptoms show[70]. Bladders issues usually are mild in the beginning but can progress to full incontinence if not treated early enough[71].

Treatment or Not Treated

If one sees a competent doctor soon enough, and he or she sends you to the right neurologist, there is a chance of recovery.

However, if one does not seek early treatment, the

condition grows progressively worse and, at some point, becomes irreversible[72].

The best option is to document symptoms, get to a doctor, provide the doctor every detail possible to help diagnosis. If the doctor diagnoses NPA early, they can treat and hopefully reverse the symptoms.

Do not allow NHP to progress past the first stage without seeing a neurologist!

IV. NORMAL PRESSURE HYDROCEPHALUS RISK FACTORS

Altogether, we uncovered 53 risk factors that increase the chances of at least one form of dementia.

Let's now break the list into two categories:

1. Uncontrollable risk factors
2. Controllable risk factors.

Chapter 8: NORMAL PRESSURE HYDROCEPHALUS RISK FACTORS

What are the risk factors for normal pressure hydrocephalus?

We need more research to confirm, normal pressure hydrocephalus risk factors include:

- Age 60 or over[73]
- Brain infections[74]
- Brain surgery history[75]
- Brain tumors[76]
- Head injuries[77]
- Hemorrhages[78]
- Inflammation[79]

Age

Age is one of a handful of symptoms that raise our risks for almost every type of dementia.

A Department of Molecular Neuroscience, Institute of Neurology, University College London concluded: "The greatest risk factor for Alzheimer's disease is advanced age[80]."

What is true for Alzheimer's is often true for the other dementias. Advancing age is a risk factor for at least 14 primary dementias.

The older we get, the more at risk we are for dementia and all adult diseases. Aging itself, however, does not lead to dementia or memory loss[81].

As we soon discuss, there is real age and birth age. While you cannot change your birth age, you must lower your real age to achieve healthy longevity.

Not counting the early-onset dementias, most people get dementia when they are 60 or older. Nature does not conspire against age, but instead, the accumulative effect of our bad habits and genetic flaws catches up with us.

Let's list the dementias science confirms age increases risks:

1. Dementia with Lewy bodies
2. Parkinson's disease dementia
3. Corticobasal syndrome
4. Normal pressure hydrocephalus
5. Wernick-Korsakoff syndrome
6. Amyotrophic lateral sclerosis
7. Typical Alzheimer's disease
8. Posterior cortical atrophy
9. Limbic-predominant Age-related TDP-43 Encephalopathy (LATE)
10. Down syndrome with AD
11. Progressive supranuclear palsy

12. Cortical Vascular Dementia
13. Binswanger disease
14. Creutzfeldt-Jakob disease (CJD)

Age increases risks for all dementia except where it likes them young. Genetics causes Huntington's disease. Early-onset Alzheimer's disease strikes when people are a bit younger in their prime, leaving three unaccounted dementias, either having no link to advanced age or science has not yet conducted the studies to confirm the connection.

Science confirms age increases risks for 14 of 19 primary dementias. However, not everybody ages the same.

Healthy and Unhealthy Habits/Real Age and Birth Age

Studies show one's normal pressure hydrocephalus risks increase as we grow older, especially once hitting sixty.

However, there is birth age and real age.

Birth Age

Birth age is beyond our control. We are born, and the clock starts ticking.

Real Age

Although physics sets our birth age in stone, our real age is rarely the same. Our real age is either older or younger than our birth age.

Habits determine the real age. What we eat, how much we exercise, and how well we sleep. Our body mass and how much visceral fat we carry. How much we read and exercise our minds. If and how much we drink alcohol. If we use tobacco products or if we tolerate them secondhand. We control if we abuse illicit, over the counter, and prescription drugs. For most of us, our lifestyle choices determine our blood pressure, blood sugar, cholesterol, and other important measurements.

Practicing healthy habits lowers our real age, while unhealthy habits make us age faster than our birth age.

Everything else we discuss, from factors beyond our

v. DIAGNOSIS & TREATMENT

Almost 50 years after the original description of NPH, there remain many unknowns, including its diagnostic criteria —
Hydrocephalus Association

Chapter 9: HOW DO DOCTORS DIAGNOSE NORMAL PRESSURE HYDROCEPHALUS?

Diagnosing normal pressure hydrocephalus frustrates health professionals, patients, and loved ones. One stands a far better chance of winning a coin toss than receiving an accurate normal pressure hydrocephalus diagnosis.

The Alzheimer's Association[82] laments over doctors misdiagnosing 80% of normal pressure hydrocephalus cases[83].

The Hydrocephalus Association[84] considers the diagnosis criteria inadequate. As evidence, they point out how medical professionals too often misdiagnose normal pressure hydrocephalus for Parkinson's disease, Alzheimer's disease, or another neurological disorder[85].

If misdiagnosed for Alzheimer's, medical authorities consider the person incurable.

Early and correct diagnosis is crucial. One of the reversible dementias, an early and correct normal pressure hydrocephalus diagnosis, is often the difference between life and death, tolerable and unbearable.

With No Accurate, Cheap, Or Quick Test, How Do Doctors Diagnose Normal Pressure Hydrocephalus?

We refer to the under 20% when doctors make the correct diagnosis, not 80% of the time they get it wrong.

To reach a correct diagnosis:

One, primary physicians and health professionals must receive better dementia training in all 19 primary dementias and their subtypes.

Two, primary physicians must refer patients to the right neurologists and others who specialize in normal pressure hydrocephalus.

Three, the specialists must:

- recognize the symptoms (Gait deterioration)
- run CAT scans and MRI's
- order cerebrospinal fluid tests
- order neuropsychological testing

If all this happens, and the neurologist ties the different signs together, he or she will make the correct diagnosis.

Let's view the normal pressure hydrocephalus diagnosis criteria.

Normal Pressure Hydrocephalus Diagnosis Criteria

A three-step process guides the diagnosis criteria[86].

1. **Clinical Examination**[87] confirms gait disturbance[88] and urinary urgency/incontinence[89], or dementia related cognitive decline[90].
2. **Brain imaging tests**[91] (CT scan[92] and/or MRI[93]) confirming hydrocephalus defined by the >30 Evans' ratio[94].
3. **Cerebrospinal fluid test**[95] predicts "shunt[96] responsiveness and/or determine shunt pressure include lumbar puncture, external lumbar drainage, measurement of CSF outflow resistance, intracranial pressure[97] (ICP) monitoring, and isotopic cisternography[98]."

Tests Doctors use to Diagnose Normal Pressure Hydrocephalus?

According to the Cleveland Clinic, there are four primary tests to diagnose normal pressure hydrocephalus[99].

- Imaging tests
- Gait analysis
- Cerebrospinal fluid tests
- Neuropsychological testing

Imaging Tests

- CT Scan
- MRI

MRI and CT scans support a clinical diagnosis by confirming "enlarged lateral and third ventricles out of proportion to the cortical sulcal enlargement[100]."

Gait Analysis

Medical authorities measure gait problems and compare the symptoms to those most prevalent in normal pressure hydrocephalus.

Medical authorities can tell much about our bones, muscles, and ligaments by how we walk.

Gait analysis measures two elements; the stance phase when both feet are secure to the ground and the swing phase when one foot is off the ground.

Gait Measurements

The analysis covers a wide range of gait-related motion. To distinguish between medical conditions such as Parkinson's disease and normal pressure hydrocephalus,

They examine cadence (rhythm), velocity, distance, autonomy (maximum walking time), routes, angles, width, momentum, posture, angles of feet, knees, legs, arms, upper body, neck, and head when walking.

Medical authorities also measure stop duration to determine gait severity and endurance.

Other Gait Measurements

- Gait phases
- Ground reaction forces
- How much electrical activity muscles produce
- Leg segment direction
- Maintaining gait over long periods
- Long step length (distance between steps of both feet)
- Short step time
- Short step stride (distance between two successive steps by same foot)
- Swing time (the time it takes each foot to lift the floor until touching again)
- Support time for each foot (when the heel touches the floor until lifting toes)
- Uneven terrain covered (height difference between drops and rises)

Sources: *ScienceDirect*[101], *PubMed*[102], Forbes[103], Temple University School of Podiatric Medicine[104], Cleveland Clinic Lerner Research Institute[105], Johns Hopkins Medicine[106]

Specialists also watch for falls and tremors while walking. They measure everything conceivable because combinations of symptoms point medical professionals toward diagnosis.

Specialists use two gait analysis types.

1. Model-based methods
2. Motion-based methods

Model-based Methods

The model-based method uses math to measure the motion of one's body parts, including the arms, legs, head, neck, and waste through segmented images.

In 2007, Mark Nixon and Imed Bouchrika from the University of Southampton, UK developed the human model-based analysis[107].

> *We propose a new approach to extract human joints (vertex positions) using a model-based method. Motion templates describing the motion of the joints, as derived by gait analysis, are parametrized using the elliptic Fourier descriptors. The heel strike data is exploited to reduce the dimensionality of the parametric models. People walk normal to the viewing plane, as major gait information is available in a sagittal view. The ankle, knee, and hip joints are successfully extracted with high accuracy for indoor and outdoor data. In this way, we have established a baseline analysis which can be deployed in recognition, marker-less analysis, and other areas.*

How Accurate Are The Tests?

The authors concluded the tests "confirmed the robustness of the proposed method to recognize walking subjects with a correct classification rate[108].

Motion-based methods

Motion-based methods extract features from image sequences.

Hidden Morkov Models

A hidden Markov model uses new devices such as smart shoes to examine gait motions and phases by getting ground contact forces[109].

Gait Energy Image

In 2005, the University of California researchers released a new spatio-temporal gait representation, which they named Gait Energy image to "characterize human walking properties for individual recognition by gait[110]."

Addressing inadequate training templates, the team also proposed[111]:

> *A novel approach for human recognition by combining statistical gait features from real and synthetic templates. We directly compute the real templates from training silhouette sequences, while we generate the synthetic templates from training sequences by simulating silhouette distortion. We use a statistical approach for learning effective features from real and synthetic templates. We compare the proposed GEI-based gait recognition approach with other gait recognition approaches on USF Human ID Database. Experimental results show that the proposed GEI is an effective and efficient gait representation for individual recognition, and the proposed approach achieves highly competitive performance with respect to the published gait recognition approaches.*

Cerebrospinal Fluid Tests

Medical professionals use cerebrospinal fluid tests to predict shunt effectiveness in patients clinically diagnosed with normal pressure hydrocephalus.

Cerebrospinal Fluid

A clear liquid, cerebrospinal fluid surrounding and protecting our central nervous system (brain and spinal cord). The U.S. National Library of Medicine explains how the central nervous system controls almost everything we consider us, and cerebrospinal fluid's role[112].

> *Your central nervous system controls and coordinates everything you do, including muscle movement, organ function, and even complex thinking and planning. CSF (cerebrospinal fluid) helps protect this system by acting like a cushion against sudden impact or injury to the brain or spinal cord. CSF also removes waste products from the brain and helps your central nervous system work properly.*

Medical authorities favor the lumbar puncture (spinal tap) to test cerebrospinal fluid, but there are other options such as fluoroscopy, cisternal puncture, and ventricular puncture[113].

Medical professionals check to see if there is too much cerebrospinal fluid surrounding and placing pressure on the brain.

The test is important for two reasons:

1. To diagnose normal pressure hydrocephalus.
2. To predict how effective a ventriculoperitoneal shunt might be in treating cerebrospinal fluid pressure.

"When spinal fluid builds up in the ventricles, it causes them to enlarge and stretch the brain tissue," explained NYU

Langone Health. "This can lead to problems with walking, cognitive impairment—such as memory problems and dementia—and diminished bladder control[114]."

Neuropsychological Testing

Many gait analysis commercial wearable sensors are on the market today, each collecting gait analysis for runners, athletes, and those suffering gait-related medical problems.

The Department of Neurosurgery, University of Cambridge School of Clinical Medicine, described neuropsychological testing's importance[115].

> *Clinical neuropsychology provides a means of determining a cognitive profile for NPH, assisting in differential diagnosis, tracking the disorder's progression, and assessing the efficacy of treatment. This article will review possible applications of clinical neuropsychology and propose a clinical assessment protocol for NPH.*

Chapter 10: TREATMENT FOR NORMAL PRESSURE HYDROCEPHALUS

Medical professionals can treat normal pressure hydrocephalus in the early stages, but the success rate drops as the medical condition progresses[116].

According to the Hydrocephalus Association, only one of five people with normal pressure hydrocephalus receive the correct treatment[117], tragic considering normal pressure hydrocephalus is one of the few dementias doctors can reverse.

A key to reversal is early diagnosis, but officials misdiagnose 80% of cases and fail to treat 4 of 5 normal pressure hydrocephalus sufferers.

Once again, I stress the need for more research funds for normal pressure hydrocephalus.

Pacific Adult Hydrocephalus Center[118] suggests two treatment forms[119].

1. Lumbar puncture
2. Ventriculoperitoneal shunt

Lumbar Puncture (Spinal Tap)

The lumbar puncture, also known as a spinal tap, helps doctors diagnose normal pressure hydrocephalus[120], but also is one of two primary treatments (the other is the ventriculoperitoneal shunt).

If the procedure provides relief, this indicates normal pressure hydrocephalus. Besides helping diagnose normal pressure hydrocephalus, medical professionals use the lumbar puncture to provide pain relief.

A neurosurgeon performs a lumbar puncture in the lower back in the lumbar area, inserting a needle between the vertebrae to collect a cerebrospinal fluid sample[121].

Although the cerebrospinal fluid protects the brain and spinal cord, an excess amount places pressure on the brain and causes the symptoms associated with normal pressure hydrocephalus[122].

The lumbar puncture measures cerebrospinal fluid pressure[123].

Lumbar Puncture Side Effects

According to the Mayo Clinic, the procedure poses the following risk factors[124]:

- Back pain (pain might include back of legs)
- Bleeding (rare)
- Brainstem herniation (when a brain tumor is present)
- Headaches (up to 25 percent)

Ventriculoperitoneal Shunt

Ventriculoperitoneal shunts are the primary form of treating normal pressure hydrocephalus.

Neurosurgeons implant ventriculoperitoneal shunts to drain excess cerebrospinal fluid from the brain. The shunt comes in three parts[125].

- The ventricular catheter
- A valve regulating cerebrospinal fluid
- A catheter running into the abdominal space

The neurosurgeon scalps an incision in the back of the head and drills a hole into the skull[126]. Inside the enlarged ventricle, the neurosurgeon passes the catheter through the brain.

A neurosurgeon inserts a shunt valve through an incision behind the ear and attaches the ventricular catheter[127].

A surgeon team makes a third incision in the belly and form a tunnel from the ear, down the chest to the abdominal. The system pumps excess cerebrospinal fluid from the brain to the belly[128], which absorbs and disperses the excess fluid.

The procedure helps many with the gait and continence problems, but Johns Hopkins Medicine warns shunts do not relieve dementia symptoms[129].

"Most types of dementia (e.g., Alzheimer's dementia) cannot be cured, but only temporized," according to Pacific Adult Hydrocephalus Center. "There are very few types of reversible dementia—one of these is Normal Pressure Hydrocephalus. Normal pressure hydrocephalus is rare dementia; the medical profession can sometimes reverse. If you show symptoms, see a doctor (neurologist). The sooner you do, the greater chance of preventing the medical condition from destroying your life and leading to premature death."

If you have normal pressure hydrocephalus symptoms, please see a doctor (neurologist) as soon as possible.

VI. BONUS SECTION

Whether diagnosed with dementia or preparing for a rainy day, there are basics everybody should consider.

This section focuses on steps dementia patients (all adults) should address, including forming a care team and understanding various therapy.

While written for dementia patients, I recommend every adult fulfill these tasks before you turn thirty. Waiting is our enemy for these two duties. Be prepared!

The section includes:

1. A starter to-do list for any adult diagnosed with a fatal disease such as dementia.
2. A care team plan.

Chapter 11: Starter To-do List for Somebody and Family once Diagnosed with Dementia.

Dementia patients, loved ones, and family must address several matters early in the disease, including care, financial decisions, living quarters, Living Will, and Power of Attorney.

While you have full or most of your cognitive skills, take care of the listed priorities before diagnosis or when diagnosed. Please do not consider the items covered in this section a complete care list, but a start you tailor to your needs.

Fail to cross these items off the list while you maintain your facilities causes much regret for patients and loved ones.

Your life is your ship, and for now, you remain the captain. Plan how your ship faces the coming storm and, when you can no longer captain the ship yourself, have it already determined who takes over the helm.

Now remains your last best chance to have a substantial say in your future.

Care

Family, loved ones, and dementia patients must make difficult decisions concerning if somebody can become the primary volunteer caregiver. While dementia patients do not require 24/7 care in the early stage, it becomes necessary in the middle to late stages.

Nobody can get through dementia without others providing years of caregiving. While rare dementias kill in months, most dementia patients live for 5-20 years, with dementia growing progressively worse.

Diagnosed with dementia or in perfect health, we all must ask ourselves who would take care of us if dementia or another devastating disorder struck, requiring longterm caregiving.

Most families cannot afford professional caregiving, and the government will not help until towards the end, so family and loved ones must.

In an ideal world, we ask ourselves these tough questions and have a plan in place should something happen. This benefits not only those diagnosed with dementia but also the heroic voluntary caregivers who will see them to the end.

Financial Decisions

There are significant financial decisions to make, and earlier, the better.

Find out how much your insurance covers and the amount you must pay. A kinder world would not burden dementia patients, nor their loved ones, with overwhelming medical care costs.

In the United States and most countries in the world, the majority of dementia costs fall on families.

How Much Does Dementia Cost The Average Family?

With no urine or blood test for most dementia types, neurologists must rely on imaging and other expensive tests, often not to diagnose dementia but to rule out other neurological disorders.

Under the best scenario, related tests, doctor visits saddle the average patient with tens of thousands of dollars in deductibles by the time the neurological team diagnoses them with dementia. For some, such as dementia with Lewy bodies, it might run much higher as it can take up to eighteen months or longer before doctors make a correct diagnosis.

Our health system tells the average person: "Sorry, you have dementia. Oh, by the way, there's the bill."

Doctors, medical professionals, hospitals, drug companies, and others involved in treating dementia must make a living. Even when we factor out overcharging and profiteering, treating dementia would remain expensive.

The average American family's health insurance has deteriorated for years, the premiums growing too high, the deductibles unaffordable, and too many not worth the paper its written, much less the monthly premiums.

Authorities estimate the average cost per dementia patient is $341,840, with families expected to cover 70 percent.

Such a disease becomes a hardship for not only the patient but also their family. The demands, financial and otherwise, on voluntary caregivers often is devastating. Make difficult financial decisions early.

Financial costs vary from one dementia to another and the treatment plan.

Living Quarters

While most dementia patients maintain independence in stage one, at some point, they require help with daily tasks. Will somebody moves in with her or him? Does the patient move in with somebody else? Will it become necessary for him or her to move into an assisted living community in later stages? If so, what type?

The person diagnosed should gather loved ones and decide such matters in the beginning. Like somebody on a small island with a hurricane approaching, one must be diligent. While no man or woman can withstand such a storm, they still take precautions to protect themselves and their families.

In part because of financial considerations, most families care for the loved one in the home until symptoms grow critical. Whether a dementia patient ends up in a special needs living facility is not a matter of if, but at what point for those who have access.

No matter how much love, care, and attention a voluntary caregiver or loved ones provide a dementia patient, they are ill-equipped to provide for somebody in the disorder's final stretch.

Families without access do the best they can to provide comfort for the loved one but make no mistake, the patient and family benefit if a special needs facility takes over at some point.

Which type of facility depends on which dementia and symptoms. Some dementias cause more cognitive problems, while others greater affect motor skills, some visual, and a few dementias cause more language problems. In the end, many dementias are more alike than not, as the damage to the brain spreads to other areas. Still, depending on the symptoms, different care facilities might be better than others.

Ask your neurologist or local dementia organizations about local facilities trained for your particular type. Hopefully, you live at home and maintain a normal or semi-normal life for years, but have a facility selected when the end grows near.

Living Will

Not to be confused with a Last Will and Testament that distributes assets, a living will focus on medical decisions. NOLO defines a living will.

> *A living will – sometimes called a health care declaration -- is a document in which you describe the kind of health care you want to receive if you are incapacitated and cannot speak for yourself. It is often paired with a power of attorney for health care, in which you name an agent to make health care decisions on your behalf. Some states combine these two documents into one document called an 'advanced directive.'*

It is crucial to document the dementia patient's wishes while you maintain facilities to make such decisions.

Use the Living Will to direct physicians to follow your wishes on what care you receive now and in the future when you might not maintain your cognitive skills.

Specify end-of-life medical treatment.

NOLO recommends prioritizing life-prolonging medical care, food, and water if you become unconscious, and palliative care, which we soon address[130].

Distribute copies of your living will to loved ones, doctors, insurance providers, and all health care facilities.

Power of Attorney

The American Bar Association describes a power of attorney:

> *A power of attorney gives one or more persons the power to act on your behalf as your agent. The power may be limited to a particular activity, such as closing the sale of your home or be general in its application. The power may give temporary or permanent authority to act on your behalf. The power may take effect immediately, or only upon the occurrence of a future event, usually a determination that you are unable to act for yourself due to mental or physical disability. The latter is called a "springing" power of attorney. A power of attorney may be revoked, but most states require written notice of revocation to the person named to act for you*[131].

It is important to establish a medical power of attorney to empower a trusted loved one to make medical decisions when a patient becomes incapable. If you do not choose the right person, you can almost count on the wrong people making important decisions down the road.

If you're in early stages dementia and reading this, you likely can still think clearly, but this changes as the symptoms worsen. The only way to protect a dementia patient's wishes when they lose their cognitive decisionmaking is by naming a power of attorney in advance.

Once you name a power of attorney, cover some dos and don'ts. After all, you are trusting another person with your life. Like with your doctors, speak your mind while you can and let people know what you expect.

As NOLO pointed out, some states merge the living will and power of attorney into an advanced directive. Whether together or separate, I recommend all adults, and particularly those diagnosed with dementia draw up a medical living will and name a power of attorney.

The starter to-do list provides a starting point for dementia patients, families, and any adult.

Once diagnosed, both the person diagnosed and loved ones must unite and build your to-do list. Add whatever makes sense for you and your unique situation.

Let's next cover a few key members of a dementia care team.

Chapter 12: CARE TEAM

The National Institute on Aging recommends building a care team.

The team includes an art therapist, mental health counselor, occupational therapist, palliative care specialist, physical therapist, and a speech therapist[132].

Art therapist

The art therapist reduces stress by engaging the patient in music and other expressive arts.

Since dementia causes enormous anxiety and mood swings, art therapists use music and art to soothe patients and assist caregivers. Most everybody responds to music. Some pump our blood and makes us want to shake our bodies to the rhythm. Other music helps us focus and achieve maximum concentration.

Some music geared towards dementia patients relaxes and calms. Music is a godsend!

Art is not a task but a love affair. Some say within each of us is an artist starving to escape. Art therapists use music and art as a brilliant tool to treat dementia anxiety, attention decline, sleep problems, etc.

Mental health counselors

A neurological disorder, dementia attacks the brain and inhibits cognitive skills. Mental health counselors help patients and families plan for the future and cope with the shock, hurt, and pain resulting from the diagnosis.

Most individuals and families suffer chronic mental stress when doctors diagnose a member with dementia.

Find a mental health counselor trained in dementia.

Turn to their expertise and do not allow the neurological disorder to destroy the remaining quality of life for the patient, or respond as a family in a way where dementia destroys many lives by one sweeping event.

Occupational therapists

The occupational therapist helps patients bathe, dress, eat, and perform daily tasks.

We think of the routine daily tasks as second nature, and it is as long as the neurons, pathways, arteries, heart, and brain perform as normal. When suffering a stroke or neurological disorder like dementia, we quickly learn nothing is second nature anymore. Like a child, dementia patients often must relearn how to perform basic tasks.

Occupational therapists help patients remain independent and then semi-independent, as long as possible, extending the quality of life. An occupational therapist is instrumental in treating most dementias.

Palliative care specialist

The palliative care specialist minimizes symptoms from diagnosis to the end. You or a loved one need somebody who addresses symptoms as soon as they arise, so find a quality palliative care specialist.

They extend the quality of life and reduce suffering.

Physical therapists

Physical therapists help motors skills by leading patients through exercise.

Although dementia is known as a mental disorder, what affects the brain affects the body and vice versa. Find a physical therapist trained to work with your specific dementia.

If you've seen somebody suffering Parkinsonism or other neurological disorders affecting movement, you have an idea of the problems some dementias cause, even in the earliest stages.

A physical therapist helps maintain balance and strength, allowing a person to walk and move on their own. As dementia progresses, so does the physical therapist's importance.

Speech therapists

The speech therapist addresses speech and swallowing problems, issues present in early dementia symptoms for some types, and eventually becomes a problem for most dementias.

What is the value of verbalizing one's thoughts, understanding what a loved one says, and swallowing our food without choking or causing infection by sending it down the wrong pipe?

These are issues speech therapists excel. The ones I've observed are passionate about helping people retrain the mind to overcome aphasia and swallowing problems.

Find a speech (and other types of) therapist trained in treating your specific type of dementia. These different listed therapists can minimize the long nightmare following a dementia diagnosis.

Chapter 13: LETTER TO CONGRESS

DEAR U.S. CONGRESS, NATIONS OF THE WORLD, & WEALTHY HUMANS

We call on the United States and the governments of the world to spend less on war and walls and more on Alzheimer's and dementia research.

If aliens were attacking us from another planet, I presume the nations of the world would unite against a common enemy. That is what I propose now.

The enemy I refer to does not come from another planet but threatens humans no less. Alzheimer's and dementia strike an American every 68 seconds and somebody worldwide every 30 seconds.

The nations of the world can save millions of lives and billions of dollars.

We need necessary funding to:

1. Discover the exact cause (s) of Alzheimer's and other dementias.
2. Develop accurate testing for Alzheimer's and other dementias.
3. Develop a vaccine to wipe out Alzheimer's and other dementias like we did polio.

Alzheimer's and dementia grow at a rate that will destroy the economies of most countries if we do not become more proactive.

We can save trillions of dollars for future generations if we invest now in discovering the exact cause (s), a vaccine to prevent it from happening, and other steps to defeat this horrifying disease.

Alzheimer's and other dementias threaten every family in all nations.

We can do little for those with late-stage dementia, but the proposed steps might save millions of lives and trillions of dollars by diagnosing the different dementias early and treating them before they do significant damage.

Beller Health calls on politicians, corporations, and wealthy individuals to step forward to help win the war against dementia.

CONCLUSION

Thank you for reading this book. We covered a good amount of material.

Dementia is a cruel neurological disorder that robs people of their personalities, executive skills, memories, talents, language, voice, motor capabilities, and all that makes us individual humans.

Alzheimer's and Dementia

Although Alzheimer's disease (AD) is the most prevalent, we learned AD is to dementia what China is to Asia. Alzheimer's represents 60-80% of dementia, but 19 dementia types account for 99 percent.

Dementia Spares No Demographic

Dementia's reputation is known as an old folk's disease but strikes people all ages. Most dementia is not genetic, although certain types such as Huntington's disease are 100% familial.

Most Dementia is Incurable

Most dementia is incurable, but—if caught early enough—neurosurgeons can treat and sometimes reverse normal pressure hydrocephalus.

Dementia Prevalence

The first section focused on dementia as a general category. We learned 850,000 people in the UK have dementia, compared to 5.8 Americans and 50 million people worldwide.

Dementia Categories
We divided the 19 dementias into six categories:
- Lewy Body/Parkinsonism related dementias
- Alzheimer's related dementias
- Frontotemporal lobar degeneration related dementias
- Primary progressive aphasia related dementias
- Vascular dementias
- Other dementias

19 Dementia Types
Lewy Body/Parkinsonism Related Dementias
1. *Dementia with Lewy Bodies*
2. *Parkinson's Disease Dementia*
3. Corticobasal Syndrome

Alzheimer's Related Dementias
4. Typical Alzheimer's Disease
5. Posterior Cortical Atrophy
6. Down Syndrome with Alzheimer's
7. Limbic-predominant Age-related TDP-43 Encephalopathy (LATE)
8. Early-onset Alzheimer's

Frontotemporal Lobar Degeneration Related Dementias
9. *Behavioral Variant Frontotemporal Dementia*
10. Progressive Supranuclear Palsy

Primary Progressive Aphasia Related Dementias
11. *Nonfluent Primary Progressive Aphasia (nfvPPA)*

12. Logopenic Progressive Aphasia (LPA)

Vascular Dementia

13. *Cortical Vascular Dementia*
14. *Binswanger Disease*

Other Dementias

15. *Normal Pressure Hydrocephalus*
16. *Huntington's Disease*
17. *Korsakoff Syndrome*
18. *Creutzfeldt-Jakob Disease*
19. Amyotrophic Lateral Sclerosis

We examined normal pressure hydrocephalus, defining and exploring causes, prevalence, symptoms, stages, and risk factors.

THE END

Of

NORMAL PRESSURE HYDROCEPHALUS

JERRY BELLER HEALTH RESEARCH INSTITUTE

THANK YOU FOR READING

Thank you for reading the entire book. While this is not a literary work to enjoy, I hope you gained useful knowledge of posterior cortical atrophy.

If you benefitted from this book, please take a moment to share your thoughts in a review. Reader reviews help other readers make educated decisions about this book before purchasing.

Book Review link for Normal Pressure Hydrocephalus
or
https://www.amazon.com/dp/B07ZDBF68D

Look for annual updates to my health books, as I follow new studies and add any helpful information I find. Health and fitness are top priorities, and the heart and brain are my specialties.

I hope you develop the habits suggested in this book. Good luck on your health journey. Live long and prosper, my friend.

All the best,
Jerry Beller & Beller Health

BELLER HEALTH BOOKS

Beller Health Research Institute specializes in the heart and brain, and published the following Jerry Beller book series:

- Arrhythmia Series
- Vascular Disease Series
- 2020 Dementia Overview Series
- 19 Dementia Types Series

Please continue to view the books in each series.

Dementia Types, Symptoms, Stages, & Risk Factors Series

This book series is the first to cover each of the 19 primary dementia types.

1. Dementia with Lewy Bodies
2. Parkinson's Disease Dementia
3. Corticobasal Syndrome
4. Typical Alzheimer's Disease
5. Posterior Cortical Atrophy
6. Down Syndrome with Alzheimer's
7. Limbic-predominant Age-related TDP-43 Encephalopathy (LATE)
8. Early-onset Alzheimer's
9. Behavioral Variant Frontotemporal Dementia
10. Progressive Supranuclear Palsy
11. Nonfluent Primary Progressive Aphasia
12. Logopenic Progressive Aphasia
13. Cortical Vascular Dementia
14. Binswanger Disease
15. Normal Pressure Hydrocephalus
16. Huntington's Disease
17. Korsakoff Syndrome
18. Creutzfeldt-Jakob Disease
19. Amyotrophic Lateral Sclerosis

2020 Dementia Overview Series

Whereas in the *Dementia Types, Symptoms, Stages, and Risk Factors* series, each book covers a different dementia type, this series focuses on groups of dementias.

1. Dementia Types, Symptoms, & Stages
2. *Lewy Body/Parkinsonism Dementias*
3. *Vascular Dementia*
4. *Frontotemporal Dementia (FTD)*
5. Alzheimer's Related Dementias
6. *Prevent or Slow Dementia*

JERRY BELLER HEALTH RESEARCH INSTITUTE

Other Beller Health Books

You can view or purchase all Beller Health Books on Amazon at the following web address:

https://amzn.to/2TpDr8e

ABOUT THE AUTHOR

Jerry Beller is the lead author and researcher at Beller Medical Research Institute. Beller distinguished himself three times in the medical world by being the first to write and publish books on particular dementia fields.

He wrote the first book covering all 15 primary dementia types, which he since expanded to cover nineteen. Beller followed this accomplishment by writing a book on each dementia type. He broke medical ground a third time when he published the first book on the new dementia category LATE.

When the world struggled to grasp the difference between Alzheimer's disease and China, Beller explained:

Alzheimer's is only one dementia, much like China is only one country in Asia. Just as we do not want to ignore the other countries in Asia because China is the largest, nor do we want to ignore the less prevalent dementia types.

Despite his accomplishments, he remains humble. "Until we win the dementia war, I've no reason to celebrate," Beller said. "If we win the war during my lifetime, I will celebrate with a few hundred brothers and sisters around the world who share my passion. Until then, we have too much work left to worry about accolades and legacies."

When not researching dementia, Jerry enjoys life with his wife of thirty-plus years, Nicola, and their two children.

Visit Jerry Beller at:

https://bellerhealth.com

1 'What Is Dementia?', Alzheimer's Disease and Dementia <https://alz.org/alzheimers-dementia/what-is-dementia> *[accessed 18 September 2019].*

2 'What Is Dementia? Symptoms, Types, and Diagnosis', National Institute on Aging <https://www.nia.nih.gov/health/what-dementia-symptoms-types-and-diagnosis> [accessed 18 September 2019].

3 'What Is Dementia?', *Alzheimer's Society* <https://www.alzheimers.org.uk/about-dementia/types-dementia/what-dementia> [accessed 18 September 2019].

4 'Dementia' <https://www.who.int/news-room/fact-sheets/detail/dementia> [accessed 18 September 2019].

5 'Risk Factors' <https://stanfordhealthcare.org/medical-conditions/brain-and-nerves/dementia/risk-factors.html> [accessed 20 September 2019].

6 W. M. van der Flier and P. Scheltens, 'Epidemiology and Risk Factors of Dementia', *Journal of Neurology, Neurosurgery & Psychiatry*, 76.suppl 5 (2005), v2–7 <https://doi.org/10.1136/jnnp.2005.082867>.

7 Kent Allen, 'Dementia Rates to Grow for African Americans, Hispanics', *AARP* <http://www.aarp.org/health/dementia/info-2018/dementia-alzheimer-cases-grow-nonwhites.html> [accessed 20 September 2019].

8 Elizabeth Rose Mayeda and others, 'Inequalities in Dementia Incidence between Six Racial and Ethnic Groups over 14 Years', *Alzheimer's & Dementia: The Journal of the Alzheimer's Association*, 12.3 (2016), 216–24 <https://doi.org/10.1016/j.jalz.2015.12.007>.

9 'African Americans at Higher Dementia Risk than Other Racial Groups', *Reuters*, 10 March 2016 <https://www.reuters.com/article/us-health-dementia-race-u-s-idUSKCN0WC2X5> [accessed 20 September 2019].

10 Steve Ford, 'Likelihood of Dementia "Higher among Black Ethnic Groups"', *Nursing Times*, 2018 <https://www.nursingtimes.net/news/research-and-innovation/likelihood-of-dementia-higher-among-black-ethnic-groups-08-08-2018/> [accessed 21 September 2019].

11 'Dementia' <https://www.who.int/news-room/fact-sheets/detail/dementia> [accessed 21 September 2019].

[12] 'Women and Alzheimer's', *Alzheimer's Disease and Dementia* <https://alz.org/alzheimers-dementia/what-is-alzheimers/women-and-alzheimer-s> [accessed 21 September 2019].

[13] 'Dementia Facts', *Dementia Consortium* <https://www.dementiaconsortium.org/dementia-facts/> [accessed 21 September 2019].

[14] 'Dementia' <https://www.who.int/news-room/fact-sheets/detail/dementia> [accessed 21 September 2019].

[15] 'Why Is Dementia Different for Women?', *Alzheimer's Society* <https://www.alzheimers.org.uk/blog/why-dementia-different-women> [accessed 21 September 2019].

[16] Jessica L. Podcasy and C. Neill Epperson, 'Considering Sex and Gender in Alzheimer Disease and Other Dementias', *Dialogues in Clinical Neuroscience*, 18.4 (2016), 437–46 <https://www.ncbi.nlm.nih.gov/pmc/articles/PMC5286729/> [accessed 21 September 2019].

[17] 'WHO | Life Expectancy', *WHO* <http://www.who.int/gho/mortality_burden_disease/life_tables/situation_trends_text/en/> [accessed 21 September 2019].

[18] 'Products - Data Briefs - Number 328 - November 2018', 2019 <https://www.cdc.gov/nchs/products/databriefs/db328.htm> [accessed 21 September 2019].

[19] Jacqui Thornton, 'WHO Report Shows That Women Outlive Men Worldwide', *BMJ*, 365 (2019), l1631 <https://doi.org/10.1136/bmj.l1631>.

[20] 'Why Do Women Live Longer Than Men?', *Time* <https://time.com/5538099/why-do-women-live-longer-than-men/> [accessed 21 September 2019].

[21] 'Dementia' <https://www.who.int/news-room/fact-sheets/detail/dementia> [accessed 20 September 2019].

[22] 'Alzheimer's Disease: Facts & Figures', *BrightFocus Foundation*, 2015 <https://www.brightfocus.org/alzheimers/article/alzheimers-disease-facts-figures> [accessed 4 September 2019].

[23] 'Facts for the Media', *Alzheimer's Society* <https://www.alzheimers.org.uk/about-us/news-and-media/facts-media> [accessed 20 September 2019].

[24] 'Countries With The Highest Rates Of Deaths From Dementia',

WorldAtlas <https://www.worldatlas.com/articles/countries-with-the-highest-rates-of-deaths-from-dementia.html> [accessed 20 September 2019].

[25] 'World Alzheimer Report 2018 - The State of the Art of Dementia Research: New Frontiers', *NEW FRONTIERS*, 48.

[26] 'ALZHEIMERS/DEMENTIA DEATH RATE BY COUNTRY', *World Life Expectancy* <https://www.worldlifeexpectancy.com/cause-of-death/alzheimers-dementia/by-country/> [accessed 24 September 2019].

[27] 'Alzheimer Europe - Research - European Collaboration on Dementia - Cost of Dementia - Regional/National Cost of Illness Estimates' <https://www.alzheimer-europe.org/Research/European-Collaboration-on-Dementia/Cost-of-dementia/Regional-National-cost-of-illness-estimates> [accessed 26 September 2019].

[28] 'Publications | NATSEM' <https://www.natsem.canberra.edu.au/publications/?publication=economic-cost-of-dementia-in-australia-2016-2056> [accessed 22 September 2019].

[29] 'Dementia UK Report', *Alzheimer's Society* <https://www.alzheimers.org.uk/about-us/policy-and-influencing/dementia-uk-report> [accessed 22 September 2019].

[30] 'Dementia Statistics – U.S. & Worldwide Stats', *BrainTest*, 2015 <https://braintest.com/dementia-stats-u-s-worldwide/> [accessed 23 September 2019].

[31] 'Newsroom | Northwestern Mutual - 2018 C.A.R.E. Study', *Newsroom | Northwestern Mutual* <https://news.northwesternmutual.com/2018-care-study> [accessed 22 September 2019].

[32] 'ALZHEIMERS/DEMENTIA DEATH RATE BY COUNTRY'.

[33] 'Alzheimer Europe - Research - European Collaboration on Dementia - Cost of Dementia - Regional/National Cost of Illness Estimates'.

[34] 'Publications | NATSEM'.

[35] 'Dementia UK Report'.

[36] 'Dementia Statistics – U.S. & Worldwide Stats'.

[37] 'Hydro- | Definition of Hydro- in English by Oxford Dictionaries', *Oxford Dictionaries | English* <https://en.oxforddictionaries.com/definition/hydro-> [accessed 9 May 2019].

[38] '-Cephalus', *TheFreeDictionary.Com* <https://medical-dictionary.thefreedictionary.com/-cephalus> [accessed 9 May 2019].

[39] 'Hydrocephalus – Causes, Symptom and Surgical Treatments' <https://www.aans.org/> [accessed 23 November 2019].

[40] 'What Is Communicating Hydrocephalus?' <https://www.medscape.com/answers/1135286-82879/what-is-communicating-hydrocephalus> [accessed 23 November 2019].

[41] **'Hydrocephalus | Genetic and Rare Diseases Information Center (GARD) – an NCATS Program'** <https://rarediseases.info.nih.gov/diseases/6682/hydrocephalus> [accessed 18 February 2018].

[42] 'Hydrocephalus' <https://www.hopkinsmedicine.org/health/conditions-and-diseases/hydrocephalus> [accessed 23 November 2019].

[43] **'Normal Pressure Hydrocephalus | Hydrocephalus Association'** <https://www.hydroassoc.org/normal-pressure-hydrocephalus/> [accessed 18 February 2018].

[44] 'Normal Pressure Hydrocephalus (NPH)', *Cleveland Clinic* <https://my.clevelandclinic.org/health/diseases/15849-normal-pressure-hydrocephalus-nph> [accessed 10 May 2019].

[45] 'Normal Pressure Hydrocephalus (NPH)', *Cleveland Clinic* <https://my.clevelandclinic.org/health/diseases/15849-normal-pressure-hydrocephalus-nph> [accessed 9 May 2019].

[46] 'Hydrocephalus Fact Sheet | National Institute of Neurological Disorders and Stroke' <https://www.ninds.nih.gov/Disorders/Patient-Caregiver-Education/Fact-Sheets/Hydrocephalus-Fact-Sheet> [accessed 9 May 2019].

[47] Caren McHenry Martin, 'The "Reversible" Dementia of Idiopathic Normal Pressure Hydrocephalus', *The Consultant Pharmacist: The Journal of the American Society of Consultant Pharmacists*, 21.11 (2006), 888–92, 901–3.

[48] 'Facts and Stats', *Hydrocephalus Association* <https://www.hydroassoc.org/about-us/newsroom/facts-and-stats-2/> [accessed 10 May 2019].

[49] 'Causes', *Hydrocephalus Association* <https://www.hydroassoc.org/causes/> [accessed 10 May 2019].

[50] 'Normal Pressure Hydrocephalus (NPH) | AdventHealth Neuroscience Institute' <http://www.adventhealthneuroinstitute.com/programs/normal-pressure-hydrocephalus> [accessed 10 May 2019].

[51] Hiroaki Kazui, '[Cognitive impairment in patients with idiopathic normal pressure hydrocephalus]', *Brain and Nerve = Shinkei Kenkyu No Shinpo*, 60.3 (2008), 225–31.

[52] A. Berardelli and others, 'Pathophysiology of Bradykinesia in Parkinson's Disease', *Brain: A Journal of Neurology*, 124.Pt 11 (2001), 2131–46.

[53] 'Cognitive Therapy for NPH Patients | Hydrocephalus Association' <https://www.hydroassoc.org/cognitive-therapy-for-nph-patients/> [accessed 18 February 2018].

[54] 'AANS | Adult-Onset Hydrocephalus' <http://www.aans.org/Patients/Neurosurgical-Conditions-and-Treatments/Adult-Onset-Hydrocephalus> [accessed 18 February 2018].

[55] 'Hydrocephalus > Condition at Yale Medicine', *Yale Medicine* <https://www.yalemedicine.org/conditions/hydrocephalus/> [accessed 18 February 2018].

[56] 'Normal Pressure Hydrocephalus: Practice Essentials, Background, Pathophysiology', 2019 <https://emedicine.medscape.com/article/1150924-overview> [accessed 10 May 2019].

[57] 'Symptoms and Diagnosis | Hydrocephalus Association' <https://www.hydroassoc.org/symptoms-and-diagnosis-nph/> [accessed 18 February 2018].

[58] 'Normal Pressure Hydrocephalus - an Overview | ScienceDirect Topics' <https://www.sciencedirect.com/topics/neuroscience/normal-pressure-hydrocephalus> [accessed 18 February 2018].

[59] 'Normal Pressure Hydrocephalus in Adults | GPonline' <https://www.gponline.com/normal-pressure-hydrocephalus-adults/article/586761> [accessed 26 December 2019].

[60] 'SHYMA.Pdf' <http://www.hydroassoc.org/docs/SHYMA.pdf> [accessed 18 February 2018].

[61] 'Hydrocephalus – Causes, Symptom and Surgical Treatments' <https://www.aans.org/> [accessed 10 May 2019].

[62] 'Hydrocephalus (for Parents) - KidsHealth' <https://kidshealth.org/en/parents/hydrocephalus.html> [accessed 10 May 2019].

[63] 'Normal Pressure Hydrocephalus', *Child Neurology Foundation* <https://www.childneurologyfoundation.org/disorder/normal-pressure-hydrocephalus/> [accessed 10 May 2019].

[64] Harvard Health Publishing, 'Hydrocephalus', *Harvard Health* <https://www.health.harvard.edu/a_to_z/hydrocephalus-a-to-z> [accessed 10 May 2019].

[65] 'Hydrocephalus', *NORD (National Organization for Rare Disorders)* <https://rarediseases.org/rare-diseases/hydrocephalus/> [accessed 10 May 2019].

[66] 'Normal Pressure Hydrocephalus', *Johns Hopkins Medicine Health Library* <https://www.hopkinsmedicine.org/health/conditions-and-diseases/hydrocephalus/normal-pressure-hydrocephalus> [accessed 10 May 2019].

[67] 'Hydrocephalus'.

[68] 'Normal Pressure Hydrocephalus (NPH) | Mischer Houston', *Neuro*, 2013 <http://neuro.memorialhermann.org/conditions-treatments/normal-pressure-hydrocephalus/> [accessed 26 December 2019].

[69] Dr Shu-Ching Hu, 'UW NPH Team Immediate Evaluation by Our Team Can Be Arranged at 206-598-5637', 2.

[70] 'Normal Pressure Hydrocephalus in Adults | GPonline'.

[71] Gary L. Gallia, Daniele Rigamonti, and Michael A. Williams, 'The Diagnosis and Treatment of Idiopathic Normal Pressure Hydrocephalus', *Nature Clinical Practice Neurology*, 2.7 (2006), 375–81 <https://doi.org/10.1038/ncpneuro0237>.

[72] 'Normal Pressure Hydrocephalus Follow-up: Prognosis, Patient Education', 2019 <https://emedicine.medscape.com/article/1150924-followup> [accessed 26 December 2019].

[73] 'Normal Pressure Hydrocephalus'.

[74] 'Hydrocephalus Fact Sheet | National Institute of Neurological Disorders and Stroke' <https://www.ninds.nih.gov/Disorders/Patient-Caregiver-Education/Fact-Sheets/Hydrocephalus-Fact-Sheet> [accessed 18 February 2018].

[75] 'Hydrocephalus Clinical Presentation: History, Physical, Causes' <https://emedicine.medscape.com/article/1135286-clinical> [accessed 11 May 2019].

[76] 'Hydrocephalus - Symptoms and Causes - Mayo Clinic' <https://www.mayoclinic.org/diseases-conditions/hydrocephalus/symptoms-causes/syc-20373604> [accessed 11 May 2019].

[77] Krauss Joachim K. and others, 'Vascular Risk Factors and Arteriosclerotic Disease in Idiopathic Normal-Pressure Hydrocephalus of the Elderly', *Stroke*, 27.1 (1996), 24–29 <https://doi.org/10.1161/01.STR.27.1.24>.

[78] 'Normal Pressure Hydrocephalus Information Page | National Institute of Neurological Disorders and Stroke' <https://www.ninds.nih.gov/Disorders/All-Disorders/Normal-Pressure-Hydrocephalus-Information-Page> [accessed 18 February 2018].

[79] 'Normal Pressure Hydrocephalus' <http://www.mayfieldclinic.com/pe-NPH.htm> [accessed 18 February 2018].

[80] Rita Guerreiro and Jose Bras, 'The Age Factor in Alzheimer's Disease', *Genome Medicine*, 7 (2015) <https://doi.org/10.1186/s13073-015-0232-5>.

[81] '2016-Facts-and-Figures.Pdf' <https://www.alz.org/documents_custom/2016-facts-and-figures.pdf> [accessed 18 February 2018].

[82] 'Home', *Alzheimer's Disease and Dementia* <https://alz.org/> [accessed 9 May 2019].

[83] 'Normal Pressure Hydrocephalus', *Alzheimer's Disease and*

Dementia <https://alz.org/alzheimers-dementia/what-is-dementia/types-of-dementia/normal-pressure-hydrocephalus> [accessed 9 May 2019].

[84] 'Hydrocephalus Association', *Hydrocephalus Association* <https://www.hydroassoc.org/> [accessed 9 May 2019].

[85] 'Normal Pressure Hydrocephalus', *Hydrocephalus Association* <https://www.hydroassoc.org/normal-pressure-hydrocephalus/> [accessed 9 May 2019].

[86] Benito Pereira Damasceno, 'Neuroimaging in Normal Pressure Hydrocephalus', *Dementia & Neuropsychologia*, 9.4 (2015), 350–55 <https://doi.org/10.1590/1980-57642015DN94000350>.

[87] 'Clinical Examination - an Overview | ScienceDirect Topics' <https://www.sciencedirect.com/topics/medicine-and-dentistry/clinical-examination> [accessed 10 May 2019].

[88] Nir Giladi, Fay B Horak, and Jeffrey M. Hausdorff, 'Classification of Gait Disturbances: Distinguishing between Continuous and Episodic Changes', *Movement Disorders☐: Official Journal of the Movement Disorder Society*, 28.11 (2013) <https://doi.org/10.1002/mds.25672>.

[89] 'What Is Urinary Incontinence? - Urology Care Foundation' <https://www.urologyhealth.org/urologic-conditions/urinary-incontinence> [accessed 10 May 2019].

[90] 'Cognitive Impairment: A Call for Action, Now!', 4.

[91] 'Types of Brain Imaging Techniques' <https://psychcentral.com/lib/types-of-brain-imaging-techniques/> [accessed 10 May 2019].

[92] 'CT Scan - Mayo Clinic' <https://www.mayoclinic.org/tests-procedures/ct-scan/about/pac-20393675> [accessed 10 May 2019].

[93] 'MRI Exam: How to Prepare & What to Expect | UCSF Radiology' <https://radiology.ucsf.edu/patient-care/prepare/mri> [accessed 10 May 2019].

[94] M. Venkatesh, 'Evans' Index | Radiology Reference Article | Radiopaedia.Org', *Radiopaedia* <https://radiopaedia.org/articles/evans-index-1?lang=us> [accessed 10 May 2019].

[95] Sara Kieffer, 'Cerebrospinal Fluid (CSF) Leak: Johns Hopkins Skull Base Tumor Center' <https://www.hopkinsmedicine.org/neurology_neurosurgery/centers_clinics/brain_tumor/center/skull-base/types/csf-leak.html> [accessed 10 May 2019].

[96] Ian K. Pople, 'Hydrocephalus and Shunts: What the Neurologist Should Know', *Journal of Neurology, Neurosurgery & Psychiatry*, 73.suppl 1 (2002), i17–22 <https://doi.org/10.1136/jnnp.73.suppl_1.i17>.

[97] Venessa L. Pinto, Prasanna Tadi, and Adebayo Adeyinka, 'Increased Intracranial Pressure', in *StatPearls* (Treasure Island (FL): StatPearls Publishing, 2019) <http://www.ncbi.nlm.nih.gov/books/NBK482119/> [accessed 10 May 2019].

[98] 'Normal Pressure Hydrocephalus', *Alzheimer's Disease and Dementia* <https://alz.org/alzheimers-dementia/what-is-dementia/types-of-dementia/normal-pressure-hydrocephalus> [accessed 10 May 2019].

[99] 'Normal Pressure Hydrocephalus (NPH) Diagnosis and Tests', *Cleveland Clinic* <https://my.clevelandclinic.org/health/diseases/15849-normal-pressure-hydrocephalus-nph/diagnosis-and-tests> [accessed 9 May 2019].

[100] Gagandeep Singh, 'Normal Pressure Hydrocephalus | Radiology Reference Article | Radiopaedia.Org', *Radiopaedia* <https://radiopaedia.org/articles/normal-pressure-hydrocephalus?lang=us> [accessed 10 May 2019].

[101] 'Gait Analysis - an Overview | ScienceDirect Topics' <https://www.sciencedirect.com/topics/neuroscience/gait-analysis> [accessed 10 May 2019].

[102] Alvaro Muro-de-la-Herran, Begonya Garcia-Zapirain, and Amaia Mendez-Zorrilla, 'Gait Analysis Methods: An Overview of Wearable and Non-Wearable Systems, Highlighting Clinical Applications', *Sensors (Basel, Switzerland)*, 14.2 (2014), 3362–94 <https://doi.org/10.3390/s140203362>.

[103] 'Running Tech: What Is A Gait Analysis And Why Should Every Runner Have One?' <https://www.forbes.com/sites/leebelltech/2018/09/30/running-tech-what-is-a-gait-analysis-and-why-should-every-runner-have-one/#6a0f1fcf79bf> [accessed 10 May 2019].

[104] 'Gait Analysis | School of Podiatric Medicine' <https://podiatry.temple.edu/research/gait-study-center/gait-analysis> [accessed 10 May 2019].

[105] 'Medical Device Solutions - Gait Lab' <http://mds.clevelandclinic.org/Services/Gait-Lab.aspx> [accessed 10 May 2019].

[106] 'Normal Pressure Hydrocephalus'.

[107] Imed Bouchrika and Mark S. Nixon, *Model-Based Feature Extraction for Gait Analysis and Recognition*.

[108] Imed Bouchrika and Mark S. Nixon, 'Model-Based Feature Extraction for Gait Analysis and Recognition', in *Proceedings of the 3rd International Conference on Computer Vision/Computer Graphics Collaboration Techniques*, MIRAGE'07 (Berlin, Heidelberg: Springer-Verlag, 2007), pp. 150–160 <http://dl.acm.org/citation.cfm?id=1759437.1759452> [accessed 10 May 2019].

[109] J. Bae, 'Gait Analysis Based on a Hidden Markov Model', in *2012 12th International Conference on Control, Automation and Systems*, 2012, pp. 1025–29.

[110] Ju Han and Bir Bhanu, 'Individual Recognition Using Gait Energy Image', *IEEE Transactions on Pattern Analysis and Machine Intelligence*, 28.2 (2006), 316–22 <https://doi.org/10.1109/TPAMI.2006.38>.

[111] Ju Han and Bir Bhanu, 'Individual Recognition Using Gait Energy Image', *IEEE Transactions on Pattern Analysis and Machine Intelligence*, 28 (2006), 316–22 <https://doi.org/10.1109/TPAMI.2006.38>.

[112] 'Cerebrospinal Fluid' <http://neuropathology-web.org/chapter14/chapter14CSF.html> [accessed 10 May 2019].

[113] 'Cerebral Spinal Fluid (CSF) Collection: MedlinePlus Medical Encyclopedia' <https://medlineplus.gov/ency/article/003428.htm> [accessed 11 May 2019].

[114] 'Diagnosing Normal Pressure Hydrocephalus' <https://nyulangone.org/conditions/normal-pressure-hydrocephalus-in-adults/diagnosis> [accessed 11 May 2019].

[115] E. E. Devito and others, 'The Neuropsychology of Normal Pressure Hydrocephalus (NPH)', *British Journal of Neurosurgery*, 19.3 (2005), 217–24 <https://doi.org/10.1080/02688690500201838>.

[116] 'NPH Left Untreated', *Hydrocephalus Association* <https://www.hydroassoc.org/nph-left-untreated/> [accessed 11 May 2019].

[117] 'New Insights into Normal Pressure Hydrocephalus', *Hydrocephalus Association* <https://www.hydroassoc.org/new-insights-into-normal-pressure-hydrocephalus/> [accessed 9 May 2019].

[118] 'Introducing the Pacific Adult Hydrocephalus Center', *Pacific Neuroscience Institute*, 2016

<https://www.pacificneuroscienceinstitute.org/blog/hydrocephalus-related-conditions/introducing-pacific-adult-hydrocephalus-center/> [accessed 10 May 2019].

[119] 'Brain Matters: Dementia Caused By Normal Pressure Hydrocephalus Can Be Reversible', *Pacific Neuroscience Institute*, 2019 <https://www.pacificneuroscienceinstitute.org/blog/hydrocephalus/brain-matters-dementia-caused-by-normal-pressure-hydrocephalus-can-be-reversible/> [accessed 10 May 2019].

[120] 'Diagnosing Normal Pressure Hydrocephalus | Swedish Medical Center Seattle and Issaquah' <https://www.swedish.org:443/services/neuroscience-institute/our-services/hydrocephalus/normal-pressure-hydrocephalus/diagnosing-normal-pressure-hydrocephalus> [accessed 10 May 2019].

[121] Radiological Society of North America (RSNA) and American College of Radiology (ACR), 'Lumbar Puncture (Spinal Tap)' <https://www.radiologyinfo.org/en/info.cfm?pg=spinaltap> [accessed 10 May 2019].

[122] 'Lumbar Puncture | Johns Hopkins Medicine' <https://www.hopkinsmedicine.org/health/treatment-tests-and-therapies/lumbar-puncture> [accessed 10 May 2019].

[123] National Center for Biotechnology Information and others, *What Happens during a Lumbar Puncture (Spinal Tap)?* (Institute for Quality and Efficiency in Health Care (IQWiG), 2016) <https://www.ncbi.nlm.nih.gov/books/NBK367574/> [accessed 10 May 2019].

[124] 'Lumbar Puncture (Spinal Tap) - Mayo Clinic' <https://www.mayoclinic.org/tests-procedures/lumbar-puncture/about/pac-20394631> [accessed 10 May 2019].

[125] 'About Your Ventriculoperitoneal (VP) Shunt Surgery', *Memorial Sloan Kettering Cancer Center* <https://www.mskcc.org/cancer-care/patient-education/about-your-ventriculoperitoneal-vp-shunt-surgery> [accessed 10 May 2019].

[126] 'Ventriculoperitonial Shunt', *Pacific Adult Hydrocephalus Center* <https://www.pacificneuroscienceinstitute.org/hydrocephalus/treatment/shunt-procedures/ventriculoperitoneal-shunt/> [accessed 10 May 2019].

[127] 'Shunt Systems', *Hydrocephalus Association* <https://www.hydroassoc.org/shunt-systems/> [accessed 10 May 2019].

[128] Julia Cannon, 'Shunt Procedure | Johns Hopkins Medicine in

Baltimore, MD'
<https://www.hopkinsmedicine.org/neurology_neurosurgery/centers_clinics/cerebral-fluid/procedures/shunts.html> [accessed 10 May 2019].

[129] Julia Cannon, 'Shunt Procedure | Johns Hopkins Medicine in Baltimore, MD'
<https://www.hopkinsmedicine.org/neurology_neurosurgery/centers_clinics/cerebral-fluid/procedures/shunts.html> [accessed 10 May 2019].

[130] Betsy Simmons Hannibal and Attorney, 'How to Write a Living Will', *Www.Nolo.Com* <https://www.nolo.com/legal-encyclopedia/how-write-living-will.html> [accessed 21 November 2019].

[131] 'Power of Attorney'
<https://www.americanbar.org/groups/real_property_trust_estate/resources/estate_planning/power_of_attorney/> [accessed 22 November 2019].

[132] 'Treatment and Management of Lewy Body Dementia', *National Institute on Aging* <https://www.nia.nih.gov/health/treatment-and-management-lewy-body-dementia> [accessed 24 April 2019].